Fenbendazole and Cancer

A Comprehensive Guide for Patients and Families

P. Carl Mullan

DCIA Publishing LLC

CONTENTS

INTRODUCTION & CHAPTER ONE

INTRODUCTION

When Joe Tippens was given three months to live in 2016, he had exhausted conventional treatment options for his small cell lung cancer. The disease had metastasized throughout his body. His doctors offered palliative care. His family began preparing for the worst. But then something unexpected happened—something that would spark a global conversation about an unlikely compound and its potential role in cancer treatment.

Joe didn't just survive those three months. He thrived. And he attributed his remarkable recovery, in part, to a veterinary deworming medication called fenbendazole—a drug designed to treat parasites in animals, not cancer in humans.

His story, shared online, went viral. Thousands of cancer patients and their families began asking questions. Could a simple, inexpensive animal medication really have anti-cancer properties? Was this a miracle cure being suppressed by pharmaceutical companies? Or was it false hope that could distract patients from proven treatments?

This book exists because those questions deserve thorough, honest, evidence-based answers.

Why This Book, Why Now

If you're reading this, you or someone you love is likely facing cancer. Perhaps you've heard about fenbendazole through online forums, social media, or word of mouth. Maybe you're skeptical but curious. Maybe you're desperate and willing to try anything. Maybe you're simply a person who believes in exploring all options and making informed decisions about your own health.

Whatever brought you here, you deserve more than anecdotes and speculation. You deserve a comprehensive examination of what we actually know about fenbendazole and cancer—the science, the evidence, the practical realities, and yes, the limitations and unknowns.

This book is not written by a doctor or medical researcher. I am not a scientist with decades of laboratory experience. I am a researcher and writer who has spent thousands of hours diving deep into the scientific literature, speaking with patients, reviewing studies, and trying to make sense of a complex and often contradictory landscape of information.

My goal is not to convince you that fenbendazole is a miracle cure. It is not to discourage you from exploring it as an option. My goal is to provide you with the most comprehensive, balanced, and practical information available so that you can make informed decisions in consultation with your healthcare team.

What Makes Fenbendazole Different

Cancer patients have always sought alternatives and supplements alongside conventional treatment. From vitamin C infusions to cannabis oil, from specialized diets to experimental immunotherapies, the landscape of cancer treatment has always included both mainstream medicine and emerging approaches.

Fenbendazole occupies an unusual space in this landscape. It's not a newly discovered compound—it's been used safely in veterinary medicine for decades. It's not expensive or difficult to obtain. It's not promoted by a pharmaceutical company with billions in marketing dollars. And yet, there's genuine scientific research suggesting it may have anti-cancer properties.

This combination—established safety profile, low cost, accessibility, and preliminary scientific support—has made fenbendazole particularly intriguing to patients who feel failed by conventional medicine or who simply want to take a more active role in their treatment.

But intrigue and hope are not the same as evidence. And that's where this book comes in.

The Promise and the Peril

Let me be direct about something from the start: fenbendazole is not FDA-approved for cancer treatment in humans. There have been no large-scale human clinical trials. We don't have the kind of robust evidence that exists for chemotherapy, radiation, or approved immunotherapies.

What we do have is:

- Laboratory studies showing anti-cancer effects in cell cultures
- Animal studies demonstrating tumor reduction in mice
- Mechanistic research explaining how fenbendazole might work against cancer
- Anecdotal reports from patients who believe it helped them
- A safety profile established through decades of veterinary use

This is simultaneously promising and insufficient. It's enough to warrant serious investigation, but not enough to make definitive claims. It's enough to explain why patients are interested, but not enough to replace proven treatments.

Throughout this book, I will walk this line carefully. I will present the evidence that exists—both supportive and critical. I will explain the science in accessible terms. I will provide practical guidance for those who choose to explore fenbendazole. And I will consistently emphasize the importance of working with qualified healthcare providers.

Who This Book Is For

This book is written for several audiences:

Cancer patients who have heard about fenbendazole and want to understand what it is, how it might work, and whether it's worth considering as part of their treatment approach.

Family members and caregivers who are trying to support a loved one with cancer and need reliable information to help guide difficult decisions.

Healthcare providers who have patients asking about fenbendazole and want a comprehensive resource to understand what their patients are reading and considering.

Researchers and advocates interested in repurposed drugs and the potential for existing medications to be used in new ways.

Anyone interested in the intersection of conventional and alternative medicine, the process of drug discovery and approval, and how patients navigate complex medical decisions.

What You'll Find in This Book

This book is organized to take you from foundational understanding to practical application:

Part One provides the scientific background—what fenbendazole is, how it works in the body, and why researchers think it might have anti-cancer properties.

Part Two examines the current research and evidence, including laboratory studies, animal research, and the limited human data available. I present both the promising findings and the significant limitations.

Part Three offers practical guidance for patients considering fenbendazole—how to research it further, questions to ask your doctors, how it's obtained and used, dosing protocols being discussed, potential side effects, and how to monitor your response.

Part Four explores real-world experiences through case studies and patient stories, helping you understand how others have approached this decision.

Part Five provides critical analysis—the concerns, the unknowns, the reasons for caution, and the importance of maintaining realistic expectations.

Part Six looks at the bigger picture—the regulatory landscape, the economics of drug repurposing, and what the fenbendazole story tells us about cancer treatment and patient empowerment.

A Note on Medical Advice

Before we go further, I must be absolutely clear: **this book is not medical advice**. I am not a doctor. I cannot diagnose, treat, or prescribe. Nothing in this book should be interpreted as a recommendation to start, stop, or modify any medical treatment.

If you're considering fenbendazole or any other treatment approach, you must discuss it with qualified healthcare providers who know your specific medical situation. Cancer is complex. Every patient is different. What works for one person may not work for another. What's safe for one person may be dangerous for another.

This book provides information and context. Your doctors provide medical care. Both are important, but they are not the same thing.

The Bigger Questions

As we explore fenbendazole specifically, we'll also be grappling with bigger questions that affect all cancer patients:

- How do we evaluate treatments that haven't gone through traditional approval processes?
- What role should patient autonomy play in treatment decisions?

- How do we balance hope with realism?
- What happens when the pace of formal research can't keep up with patient need?
- How do we think about risk and benefit when facing a life-threatening disease?

These questions don't have simple answers. But they're worth asking, and they're worth thinking about carefully.

My Commitment to You

As you read this book, I commit to several principles:

Honesty: I will tell you what we know and what we don't know. I will not exaggerate benefits or minimize risks.

Balance: I will present multiple perspectives, including those skeptical of fenbendazole's potential.

Clarity: I will explain complex science in accessible language without dumbing it down or oversimplifying.

Practicality: I will provide actionable information you can use, not just abstract theory.

Respect: I will respect your intelligence, your autonomy, and your right to make informed decisions about your own body.

A Personal Note

I came to this topic not as a cancer patient myself, but as someone who watched a close friend navigate a cancer diagnosis. I saw her struggle with the limitations of conventional treatment. I saw her research alternatives. I saw her try to make sense of conflicting information online. I saw her doctors dismiss her questions about supplements and repurposed drugs without really engaging with the evidence.

That experience made me realize how difficult it is for patients to get reliable, comprehensive information about emerging treatments. The medical establishment often dismisses anything not FDA-approved. Alternative medicine advocates often make exaggerated claims. And patients are left in the middle, trying to separate signal from noise while facing the most important decisions of their lives.

This book is my attempt to provide what I wish had existed for my friend—a thorough, balanced, practical guide that takes both the science and the patient experience seriously.

How to Use This Book

You don't have to read this book cover to cover, though I hope you will. It's designed so you can:

- Start with the practical guidance sections if you're already familiar with the basics
- Focus on the scientific chapters if you want to understand the mechanisms
- Jump to the case studies if you learn best through stories
- Use the critical analysis section to pressure-test your thinking

Throughout the book, I've included:

- **Key Takeaways** boxes summarizing important points
- **Questions to Ask Your Doctor** to facilitate productive conversations

- **Resources** for further research
- **Caution** notes highlighting important safety considerations

The Journey Ahead

Cancer is terrifying. The uncertainty is overwhelming. The desire to do something—anything—that might help is completely understandable. But desperation can make us vulnerable to false promises and dangerous choices.

My hope is that this book will help you navigate this difficult terrain with both hope and wisdom. Fenbendazole may or may not be part of your cancer journey. But understanding it fully—its potential, its limitations, and its place in the broader landscape of cancer treatment—will help you make better decisions regardless of what path you choose.

Let's begin by understanding exactly what fenbendazole is and how it works in the body.

PART ONE: UNDERSTANDING FENBENDAZOLE

CHAPTER ONE: WHAT IS FENBENDAZOLE?

To understand whether fenbendazole might have a role in cancer treatment, we first need to understand what it is, where it comes from, and how it normally functions. This foundation will help us later grasp why researchers think it might work against cancer cells.

The Benzimidazole Family

Fenbendazole belongs to a class of drugs called benzimidazoles. These are anthelmintic medications—drugs designed to kill parasitic worms. The benzimidazole family includes several compounds you may have heard of:

- **Mebendazole**: Used in humans to treat pinworms, roundworms, and other intestinal parasites
- **Albendazole**: Another human antiparasitic, often used for more serious parasitic infections
- **Fenbendazole**: Primarily used in veterinary medicine for dogs, cats, horses, and livestock
- **Thiabendazole**: Used both in humans and animals, also has antifungal properties

All of these drugs share a similar chemical structure—a benzimidazole ring—which gives them their name and their basic mechanism of action. Understanding this family relationship is important because research on one benzimidazole often provides insights into others.

Fenbendazole's Original Purpose

Fenbendazole was developed in the 1970s by Hoechst AG (now part of Bayer) as a broad-spectrum anthelmintic for veterinary use. Its primary job is to kill parasitic worms in animals by disrupting their cellular structure.

In veterinary medicine, fenbendazole is used to treat:

- Roundworms (nematodes)
- Hookworms

- Whipworms
- Some tapeworms
- Certain protozoan parasites like Giardia

It's considered highly effective and remarkably safe in animals. Dogs, cats, horses, cattle, and other animals have been treated with fenbendazole for decades with an excellent safety record. It's available over-the-counter in many countries for pet use, which speaks to its established safety profile.

The typical veterinary use involves a short course of treatment—usually three to five days—to eliminate parasitic infections. The drug is generally well-tolerated, with few side effects in animals at recommended doses.

How Fenbendazole Works Against Parasites

To understand how fenbendazole might work against cancer, we first need to understand its original mechanism of action against parasites.

Fenbendazole works by binding to a protein called tubulin. Tubulin is a fundamental building block of cellular structure. Individual tubulin proteins link together to form microtubules—tiny tubes that serve as the cell's skeleton and highway system.

Microtubules are essential for:

- Maintaining cell shape
- Moving materials within the cell
- Cell division (mitosis)
- Cell movement

When fenbendazole binds to tubulin in parasitic worms, it prevents tubulin from forming proper microtubules. Without functional microtubules, the parasite's cells cannot maintain their structure or divide. The parasite essentially falls apart at the cellular level and dies.

Importantly, fenbendazole shows selectivity—it binds much more strongly to parasite tubulin than to mammalian tubulin. This selectivity is why it can kill worms without significantly harming the host animal. The drug concentrates in the parasite and disrupts its cellular machinery while having minimal effect on the animal's own cells.

This selectivity isn't perfect, but it's good enough that fenbendazole can be used safely in animals at doses that effectively kill parasites.

Chemical Properties and Pharmacology

Understanding fenbendazole's chemical properties helps explain how it behaves in the body:

Chemical formula: C15H13N3O2S**Molecular weight**: 299.3 5 g/mol**Appearance**: White to off-white powder**Solubility**: Poorly soluble in water, more soluble in organic solvents

The poor water solubility is significant. It means fenbendazole isn't easily absorbed from the digestive tract, which is actually advantageous for treating intestinal parasites—the drug stays in the gut where the parasites live. But it also means that when fenbendazole is used for systemic effects (like potentially treating cancer), absorption and bioavailability become important considerations.

When fenbendazole is absorbed into the bloodstream, it undergoes metabolism in the liver. The primary metabolite (breakdown product) is called oxfendazole, which also has antiparasitic activity. Both fenbendazole and its metabolites are eventually excreted, primarily through feces.

The half-life of fenbendazole in animals varies by species but is generally in the range of 10-15 hours. This means the drug is cleared from the body relatively quickly, which is why repeated dosing is necessary for sustained effects.

Why Fenbendazole Instead of Mebendazole?

You might wonder why fenbendazole has received particular attention for cancer when mebendazole is already approved for human use. This is a reasonable question, and the answer involves several factors:

Availability: Fenbendazole is readily available over-the-counter for pet use in many countries, making it accessible to patients without a prescription.

Cost: Fenbendazole is generally less expensive than mebendazole, particularly in veterinary formulations.

Research timing: Some of the early research suggesting anti-cancer effects happened to use fenbendazole, which then attracted patient attention and further research.

Joe Tippens' story: The viral nature of Joe Tippens' recovery story specifically mentioned fenbendazole, creating awareness and interest in this particular drug.

That said, mebendazole has also been studied for anti-cancer effects, and some researchers and patients prefer it precisely because it's already approved for human use. We'll discuss mebendazole more in later chapters when we examine the research.

The key point is that fenbendazole isn't necessarily superior to other benzimidazoles for cancer—it's simply the one that has received the most attention in patient communities.

Forms and Formulations

Fenbendazole is available in several forms:

Granules or powder: Often mixed with food for pets. Common brand names include Panacur and Safe-Guard.

Paste: A gel formulation used for horses, measured in syringes.

Suspension: A liquid form, also commonly used for pets.

Tablets: Less common but available in some markets.

For veterinary use, the concentration and dosing are calculated based on the animal's weight. A typical dog dose might be 50 mg per kilogram of body weight, given once daily for three days.

When patients consider using fenbendazole, they're typically using these veterinary formulations, which raises important questions about purity, dosing accuracy, and appropriateness for human use. We'll address these practical considerations in detail in Part Three.

Safety Profile in Veterinary Use

One reason fenbendazole has attracted interest for human use is its excellent safety record in animals. Decades of veterinary use have established that:

- Fenbendazole is well-tolerated at recommended doses
- Side effects are rare and usually mild (occasional vomiting or diarrhea)
- It can be used in pregnant animals (though this is sometimes avoided as a precaution)
- Overdoses are rarely serious unless extremely large amounts are consumed
- It doesn't typically interact with other medications

This safety profile is reassuring, but it's important to remember that veterinary safety doesn't automatically translate to human safety, and safety at antiparasitic doses doesn't guarantee safety at potentially higher doses that might be used for cancer.

The Leap from Veterinary to Human Use

The idea of using veterinary medications in humans might seem strange, but it's not unprecedented. Many drugs were first developed for animals and later adapted for human use, or vice versa. The biology of mammals is similar enough that drugs often work across species.

However, there are important differences:

Dosing: Animals and humans metabolize drugs differently. A safe dose for a dog isn't necessarily safe for a human of the same weight.

Purity standards: Veterinary medications may not be manufactured to the same purity standards as human pharmaceuticals.

Formulations: Veterinary products may contain inactive ingredients that are safe for animals but not tested in humans.

Regulatory oversight: Veterinary drugs don't go through the same rigorous human testing that FDA-approved human drugs undergo.

These differences don't mean veterinary fenbendazole is necessarily unsafe for humans—many people have used it without apparent harm—but they do mean we should approach its use thoughtfully and carefully.

Key Takeaways

- Fenbendazole is a benzimidazole antiparasitic drug used in veterinary medicine for decades

- It works by disrupting microtubules, which are essential for cell structure and division
- It has an excellent safety record in animals at antiparasitic doses
- It's readily available and inexpensive, which partly explains patient interest
- Its poor water solubility affects how it's absorbed and distributed in the body
- Veterinary safety doesn't automatically translate to human safety, especially at different doses

CHAPTER TWO: FROM PARASITES TO CANCER

The leap from "kills parasitic worms" to "might fight cancer" isn't as random as it might seem. There's a scientific rationale for why researchers began investigating fenbendazole's potential anti-cancer properties. Understanding this rationale is crucial for evaluating whether the interest in fenbendazole is based on solid science or wishful thinking.

The Microtubule Connection

Remember that fenbendazole works by disrupting microtubules in parasitic cells. This mechanism is significant because microtubules are also crucial for cancer cells—perhaps even more so than for normal cells.

Cancer cells divide rapidly and uncontrollably. This rapid division requires functional microtubules. During cell division (mitosis), microtubules form the mitotic spindle—the structure that pulls chromosomes apart so each daughter cell gets a complete set of genetic material.

If you disrupt microtubules, you disrupt cell division. If you disrupt cell division, you can stop cancer growth.

This isn't a new idea. In fact, some of our most successful cancer drugs work by targeting microtubules:

Taxanes (paclitaxel, docetaxel): These drugs stabilize microtubules, preventing them from breaking down. This sounds opposite to fenbendazole's mechanism, but the result is similar—disrupted cell division.

Vinca alkaloids (vincristine, vinblastine): These drugs prevent microtubule formation, similar to benzimidazoles.

Colchicine: An ancient drug derived from autumn crocus, also disrupts microtubules.

So the basic concept—disrupting microtubules to stop cancer cell division—is well-established in oncology. The question is whether fenbendazole can do this effectively in cancer cells while sparing normal cells.

Selectivity: The Cancer Cell Difference

For a microtubule-disrupting drug to be useful against cancer, it needs some degree of selectivity. It needs to affect cancer cells more than normal cells. Otherwise, it would be too toxic to use.

Cancer cells differ from normal cells in several ways that might make them more vulnerable to microtubule disruption:

Rapid division: Cancer cells divide much more frequently than most normal cells. They're constantly in the process of mitosis, making them more dependent on functional microtubules.

Checkpoint defects: Normal cells have quality control checkpoints that stop division if something goes wrong. Many cancer cells have defective checkpoints, so they try to divide even when their microtubules are disrupted, leading to cell death.

Metabolic differences: Cancer cells often have altered metabolism and may take up or process drugs differently than normal cells.

Genetic instability: Cancer cells' genetic instability might make them more sensitive to additional cellular stress.

These differences create a therapeutic window—a range of doses where cancer cells are affected more than normal cells. The question for fenbendazole is whether this window exists and whether it's wide enough to be clinically useful.

The Accidental Discovery

The story of how researchers first noticed fenbendazole's potential anti-cancer effects is instructive. It wasn't a planned investigation—it was an accident.

In the 1990s and early 2000s, researchers at Johns Hopkins and other institutions were conducting cancer research using mice. These mice were routinely treated with fenbendazole to prevent parasitic infections—standard practice in animal research facilities.

Some researchers noticed something odd: their cancer experiments weren't working as expected. Tumors that should have grown weren't growing, or were growing more slowly than in previous experiments.

After investigation, they realized the difference was the fenbendazole treatment. Mice that received fenbendazole showed reduced tumor growth compared to mice that didn't receive it.

This accidental observation led to intentional research. If fenbendazole was affecting tumor growth in mice, maybe it had anti-cancer properties worth investigating.

This type of serendipitous discovery isn't unusual in medicine. Penicillin, X-rays, and many other medical advances came from unexpected observations. But an accidental discovery is just the beginning—it needs to be followed by rigorous research to determine if the effect is real, how it works, and whether it's clinically useful.

Multiple Mechanisms of Action

As researchers investigated further, they discovered that fenbendazole's anti-cancer effects might involve more than just microtubule disruption. The drug appears to affect cancer cells through several mechanisms:

Microtubule disruption: The primary mechanism, preventing cell division.

Glucose metabolism interference: Some research suggests fenbendazole may interfere with how cancer cells process glucose (sugar). Cancer cells are often highly dependent on glucose for energy (the Warburg effect), so disrupting glucose metabolism could starve cancer cells.

P53 activation: P53 is a tumor suppressor protein often called the "guardian of the genome." It triggers cell death when cells are damaged or abnormal. Some studies suggest benzimidazoles can activate p53, potentially causing cancer cells to self-destruct.

Inhibition of cancer cell signaling: Fenbendazole may interfere with signaling pathways that cancer cells use to survive and proliferate.

Anti-inflammatory effects: Chronic inflammation can promote cancer growth. Some research suggests benzimidazoles have anti-inflammatory properties.

Antioxidant effects: Paradoxically, while some cancer treatments work by creating oxidative stress, some research suggests fenbendazole may have antioxidant properties that could protect normal cells.

Immune system modulation: Some evidence suggests benzimidazoles might enhance immune system recognition of cancer cells.

It's important to note that not all of these mechanisms are equally well-established. Some are supported by multiple studies, while others are based on preliminary research. The existence of multiple potential mechanisms is both encouraging (more ways to fight cancer) and complicating (harder to understand exactly what's happening).

The Dose Question

One critical question is whether the doses of fenbendazole that show anti-cancer effects in laboratory studies are achievable and safe in humans.

In cell culture studies (cells in a dish), researchers can expose cancer cells to specific concentrations of fenbendazole and observe the effects. These studies have shown anti-cancer effects at concentrations that seem potentially achievable in human blood.

In mouse studies, researchers can give mice specific doses of fenbendazole and measure tumor growth. These studies have also shown positive effects at doses that, when adjusted for body weight and metabolism, seem potentially translatable to humans.

However, translating doses from mice to humans isn't straightforward. Mice metabolize drugs differently than humans. They have different body surface area to weight ratios. They have different lifespans, so the duration of treatment means something different.

The doses of fenbendazole that some cancer patients use (often 222 mg daily, based on Joe Tippens' protocol) are higher than typical antiparasitic doses but lower than doses that have caused toxicity in animal studies. Whether these doses achieve sufficient concentrations in human tumors to have anti-cancer effects is unknown.

Bioavailability Challenges

Remember that fenbendazole is poorly soluble in water, which limits its absorption from the digestive tract. This is fine for treating intestinal parasites but potentially problematic for treating cancer throughout the body.

Researchers have explored ways to improve fenbendazole's bioavailability:

Taking it with fats: Fenbendazole is more soluble in fats than water, so taking it with a fatty meal may improve absorption.

Micronized formulations: Grinding fenbendazole into very fine particles increases surface area and may improve absorption.

Alternative delivery methods: Some researchers have investigated injectable or other formulations, though these aren't available to patients.

Combination with other compounds: Some substances might enhance fenbendazole absorption or effectiveness.

The bioavailability question is crucial because if fenbendazole isn't well absorbed, it might not reach tumors in sufficient concentrations to have an effect, regardless of its theoretical anti-cancer properties.

Comparison to Approved Cancer Drugs

How does fenbendazole's potential anti-cancer activity compare to approved cancer drugs?

This is difficult to answer definitively because we don't have head-to-head comparisons in humans. But we can make some observations:

Potency: In cell culture studies, fenbendazole's anti-cancer effects are generally weaker than those of approved chemotherapy drugs. It takes higher concentrations of fenbendazole to kill cancer cells than it takes of drugs like paclitaxel or doxorubicin.

Selectivity: Fenbendazole appears to have a better therapeutic window (difference between effective and toxic doses) than many chemotherapy drugs, at least in animal studies.

Spectrum of activity: Fenbendazole has shown activity against various cancer types in laboratory studies, suggesting broad-spectrum potential similar to some chemotherapy drugs.

Resistance: We don't know much about whether cancer cells can develop resistance to fenbendazole, though resistance to microtubule-targeting drugs is a known phenomenon in oncology.

The comparison suggests that fenbendazole might be less potent but potentially safer than conventional chemotherapy. Whether this trade-off is favorable depends on many factors, including cancer type, stage, and individual patient circumstances.

The Repurposing Advantage

Fenbendazole represents a category of treatment called "drug repurposing"—using existing drugs for new purposes. Drug repurposing has several potential advantages:

Known safety profile: Decades of use in animals provides safety data that would take years to generate for a new drug.

Lower cost: Fenbendazole is off-patent and inexpensive to manufacture.

Faster development: Repurposed drugs can potentially move through development faster than new drugs because some safety testing is already done.

Accessibility: Fenbendazole is already available, so patients can access it without waiting for approval.

However, repurposing also has challenges:

Lack of financial incentive: Pharmaceutical companies have little incentive to fund expensive clinical trials for off-patent drugs they can't profit from.

Dosing uncertainty: The optimal dose for cancer might be very different from the antiparasitic dose.

Formulation issues: Veterinary formulations may not be ideal for human cancer treatment.

Regulatory hurdles: Even repurposed drugs need to go through approval processes for new indications.

These challenges help explain why, despite promising preliminary research, fenbendazole hasn't advanced to large-scale human trials for cancer.

What the Laboratory Studies Show

Let's look more specifically at what laboratory research has demonstrated:

Cell culture studies: Multiple studies have shown that fenbendazole and related benzimidazoles can kill various types of cancer cells in culture, including:

- Lung cancer cells

- Colon cancer cells
- Breast cancer cells
- Prostate cancer cells
- Brain cancer cells (glioblastoma)
- Lymphoma cells

The effects are dose-dependent—higher concentrations kill more cells. The effects are also time-dependent—longer exposure produces greater cell death.

Animal studies: Research in mice has shown that fenbendazole can:

- Slow tumor growth
- Reduce tumor size
- Extend survival in some cancer models
- Enhance the effects of other cancer treatments when used in combination

These effects have been demonstrated in various cancer types, including lung cancer, lymphoma, and others.

Mechanism studies: Research has confirmed that fenbendazole:

- Disrupts microtubules in cancer cells
- Causes cell cycle arrest (stops cells from dividing)
- Triggers apoptosis (programmed cell death)
- May affect cancer cell metabolism

This body of laboratory research provides a scientific foundation for interest in fenbendazole. It's not just speculation or wishful thinking—there's real evidence that fenbendazole has anti-cancer activity in laboratory settings.

The Critical Gap: Human Studies

Here's the crucial limitation: almost all of this research has been done in cell cultures or animals, not humans.

Cell cultures are useful for understanding mechanisms and screening for activity, but they're highly artificial. Cancer cells in a dish don't behave exactly like cancer cells in a living body. They don't have a blood supply, an immune system, or the complex tissue environment of a real tumor.

Mouse studies are more relevant but still limited. Mice aren't humans. Their metabolism, immune systems, and cancer biology differ in important ways. Many drugs that work in mice fail in humans.

The progression from laboratory research to human treatment typically involves:

1. Cell culture studies (in vitro)

2. Animal studies (in vivo)

3. Phase I human trials (safety and dosing)

4. Phase II human trials (preliminary efficacy)

5. Phase III human trials (large-scale efficacy)

6. FDA approval and post-market monitoring

For fenbendazole and cancer, we have steps 1 and 2, but not 3-6. This gap is significant. It means we're extrapolating from laboratory research to human use without the clinical trial data that normally guides medical practice.

Why the Research Hasn't Advanced

Given the promising laboratory research, why hasn't fenbendazole advanced to human clinical trials for cancer?

Funding: Clinical trials are expensive—often tens or hundreds of millions of dollars. Pharmaceutical companies fund most cancer drug trials, but they have little incentive to fund trials for off-patent drugs like fenbendazole.

Academic funding: Government and foundation funding for cancer research is limited and competitive. Researchers may struggle to get funding for trials of repurposed veterinary drugs when there are many other promising approaches.

Regulatory complexity: Even for repurposed drugs, conducting formal clinical trials requires extensive regulatory approval and oversight.

Scientific conservatism: The medical research establishment tends to be conservative, focusing on novel targeted therapies and immunotherapies rather than old veterinary drugs.

Lack of commercial interest: Without patent protection, there's no clear path to profitability, which discourages investment.

This funding gap is a real problem in drug repurposing generally. Many potentially useful drugs may never be properly tested because the financial incentives don't align with the public health need.

Patient-Driven Research

Interestingly, the fenbendazole story represents a new phenomenon in medicine: patient-driven research and experimentation.

Traditionally, medical research followed a top-down model: scientists and doctors decided what to study, conducted research, and then offered treatments to patients. Patients were passive recipients of medical knowledge.

The internet has changed this dynamic. Patients now:

- Share information and experiences directly with each other
- Organize to fund research on treatments that interest them
- Experiment with treatments before formal approval
- Create pressure for research on promising but under-studied approaches

Joe Tippens' story went viral not through medical journals but through social media and online forums. Thousands of patients began trying fenbendazole based on his anecdote and the preliminary scientific research, creating a large-scale, uncontrolled, unmonitored experiment.

This patient-driven approach has both benefits and risks:

Benefits:

- Patients take active roles in their treatment
- Attention is drawn to potentially useful but under-studied treatments
- Real-world data is generated (though not in a controlled way)
- Pressure is created for formal research

Risks:

- Patients may use treatments that are ineffective or harmful
- Anecdotes may be mistaken for evidence
- Patients may delay or avoid proven treatments
- Safety issues may not be detected without proper monitoring

The fenbendazole phenomenon illustrates both the promise and the peril of patient-driven medical experimentation in the internet age.

Key Takeaways

- Fenbendazole's anti-cancer potential is based on its ability to disrupt microtubules, which cancer cells need for division
- Laboratory research shows fenbendazole can kill cancer cells and slow tumor growth in mice
- Multiple mechanisms may contribute to anti-cancer effects beyond just microtubule disruption
- The drug's poor bioavailability may limit its effectiveness in humans
- There's a significant gap between laboratory research and human clinical evidence
- Lack of funding for clinical trials is a major barrier to advancing research
- The fenbendazole story represents a new model of pa-

tient-driven medical exploration

CHAPTER THREE: THE BIOLOGY OF CANCER AND WHY MICROTUBULE DISRUPTION MATTERS

To fully understand fenbendazole's potential role in cancer treatment, we need to understand cancer itself—what it is, how it grows, and why disrupting microtubules might be an effective strategy against it.

What Is Cancer?

At its most basic, cancer is a disease of uncontrolled cell growth. But this simple definition masks enormous complexity.

Normal cells in your body follow strict rules:

- They divide only when needed

- They stay in their designated locations
- They perform their specialized functions
- They die when they're damaged or old

Cancer cells break these rules:

- They divide uncontrollably
- They invade other tissues
- They lose their specialized functions
- They resist signals to die

Cancer isn't one disease—it's hundreds of diseases with different causes, behaviors, and treatments. Lung cancer is different from breast cancer, which is different from leukemia. Even within one cancer type, there's enormous variation. Two people with "breast cancer" may have tumors with completely different genetic profiles and treatment responses.

This diversity is important when evaluating any potential cancer treatment, including fenbendazole. A treatment that works for one cancer type might not work for another.

The Hallmarks of Cancer

Cancer researchers have identified several key characteristics that most cancers share, called the "hallmarks of cancer":

Sustained proliferative signaling: Cancer cells generate their own growth signals or become hypersensitive to normal growth signals.

Evading growth suppressors: Cancer cells ignore signals that normally stop cell division.

Resisting cell death: Cancer cells avoid apoptosis (programmed cell death) that would normally eliminate damaged cells.

Enabling replicative immortality: Normal cells can only divide a limited number of times. Cancer cells bypass this limit.

Inducing angiogenesis: Cancer cells stimulate the growth of new blood vessels to supply the tumor with nutrients and oxygen.

Activating invasion and metastasis: Cancer cells gain the ability to invade surrounding tissues and spread to distant sites.

Reprogramming energy metabolism: Cancer cells alter their metabolism to support rapid growth.

Evading immune destruction: Cancer cells develop ways to hide from or suppress the immune system.

Understanding these hallmarks helps us evaluate potential treatments. An effective cancer treatment needs to interfere with one or more of these hallmarks.

Where Microtubule Disruption Fits

Microtubule-disrupting drugs like fenbendazole primarily target the first hallmark: sustained proliferative signaling. By preventing cell division, they directly attack cancer's fundamental characteristic—uncontrolled growth.

But microtubule disruption may also affect other hallmarks:

Resisting cell death: When cells can't complete division properly due to microtubule disruption, they may trigger apoptosis. This could help overcome cancer cells' resistance to death.

Invasion and metastasis: Microtubules are involved in cell movement. Disrupting them might reduce cancer cells' ability to invade and metastasize.

Angiogenesis: Some research suggests microtubule-disrupting drugs may interfere with the formation of new blood vessels.

This multi-faceted impact is part of why microtubule-targeting drugs have been successful in cancer treatment.

The Cell Cycle and Cancer

To understand why rapidly dividing cancer cells are particularly vulnerable to microtubule disruption, we need to understand the cell cycle—the process by which cells divide.

The cell cycle has several phases:

G1 phase: The cell grows and prepares for DNA replication.

S phase: DNA is replicated, so the cell has two copies of its genetic material.

G2 phase: The cell continues growing and prepares for division.

M phase (mitosis): The cell divides into two daughter cells.

G0 phase: A resting state where cells aren't actively dividing.

Most normal cells in your body are in G0—they're not dividing. They only enter the cell cycle when needed (for example, to replace damaged cells or during growth).

Cancer cells, in contrast, are constantly cycling. They're always in G1, S, G2, or M phase, rarely resting in G0.

Microtubule-disrupting drugs primarily affect M phase—the actual division process. When cancer cells try to divide but can't because their microtubules are disrupted, they either:

- Arrest in M phase and eventually die

- Try to complete division abnormally and die from the resulting damage

- Trigger apoptosis in response to the mitotic failure

Because cancer cells divide much more frequently than most normal cells, they spend more time in M phase and are therefore more vulnerable to microtubule-disrupting drugs.

Why Some Normal Cells Are Also Affected

If microtubule-disrupting drugs primarily affect dividing cells, why do they cause side effects?

The answer is that some normal cells do divide frequently:

Bone marrow cells: Constantly producing new blood cells. This is why chemotherapy often causes low blood counts.

Hair follicle cells: Rapidly dividing to produce hair. This is why chemotherapy often causes hair loss.

Gastrointestinal lining cells: The lining of your digestive tract is constantly being renewed. This is why chemotherapy often causes nausea, diarrhea, and mouth sores.

Reproductive cells: Sperm and egg production involves rapid cell division. This is why chemotherapy can affect fertility.

These side effects are the price of targeting rapidly dividing cells. The hope with any microtubule-disrupting drug, including fenbendazole, is that the therapeutic window is wide enough—that cancer cells are affected at doses that don't cause intolerable side effects in normal tissues.

Tumor Heterogeneity: Why Cancer Is So Hard to Treat

One of the biggest challenges in cancer treatment is tumor heterogeneity—the fact that not all cells within a tumor are identical.

A single tumor may contain:

- Cells dividing rapidly
- Cells dividing slowly or not at all
- Cells with different genetic mutations
- Cells with different drug sensitivities
- Cancer stem cells that can regenerate the tumor

This heterogeneity means that a treatment that kills most cancer cells might miss some, allowing the tumor to regrow. It's one reason why combination therapies (using multiple drugs with different mechanisms) are often more effective than single drugs.

For fenbendazole, this heterogeneity raises important questions:

- Will it affect all cells in a tumor or only rapidly dividing ones?
- Will slowly dividing cancer cells or cancer stem cells be resistant?
- Would it need to be combined with other treatments to be fully effective?

The Tumor Microenvironment

Cancer cells don't exist in isolation. They're surrounded by a complex environment called the tumor microenvironment, which includes:

Blood vessels: Supplying nutrients and oxygen**Immune cells**: Which may attack the tumor or be suppressed by it**Fibroblasts**: Cells that produce structural proteins**Extracellular matrix**: The structural scaffolding between cells**Signaling molecules**: Chemical signals that affect cell behavior

This microenvironment profoundly influences how cancer cells behave and how they respond to treatment. Some areas of a tumor may have good blood supply and oxygen (well-perfused), while other areas may be oxygen-poor (hypoxic). Drugs may not penetrate well into poorly perfused areas.

For fenbendazole to be effective, it needs to:

- Reach cancer cells throughout the tumor
- Achieve sufficient concentrations in the tumor microenvironment
- Maintain those concentrations long enough to have an effect

The tumor microenvironment is one reason why drugs that work well in cell culture (where cells are in a uniform, well-oxygenated environment) may work less well in actual tumors.

Cancer Metabolism and the Warburg Effect

Cancer cells have altered metabolism compared to normal cells. Most notably, they exhibit what's called the Warburg effect—they preferentially use glycolysis (breaking down glucose without oxygen) for energy, even when oxygen is available.

Normal cells use glycolysis only when oxygen is scarce. When oxygen is available, they use a more efficient process called oxidative phosphorylation. Cancer cells, oddly, use glycolysis even when oxygen is present.

Why would cancer cells use a less efficient energy process? Several theories exist:

- Glycolysis produces building blocks for rapid cell growth
- It allows cancer cells to survive in low-oxygen environments
- It may help cancer cells evade the immune system

This altered metabolism is relevant to fenbendazole because some research suggests benzimidazoles may interfere with cancer cell glucose metabolism. If fenbendazole disrupts both microtubules and glucose metabolism, it could hit cancer cells with a one-two punch.

Drug Resistance: Cancer's Adaptation

One of the biggest challenges in cancer treatment is drug resistance. Cancer cells can develop resistance to drugs through various mechanisms:

Increased drug efflux: Cancer cells may pump drugs out faster, reducing intracellular concentrations.

Target mutations: The drug's target (like tubulin) may mutate so the drug no longer binds effectively.

Alternative pathways: Cancer cells may activate alternative survival pathways that bypass the drug's effect.

Reduced drug activation: If a drug needs to be activated in the cell, cancer cells may lose the enzymes that activate it.

Increased DNA repair: Cancer cells may enhance their ability to repair drug-induced damage.

For microtubule-targeting drugs, resistance often involves:

- Mutations in tubulin that reduce drug binding

- Overexpression of drug efflux pumps
- Changes in microtubule dynamics

We don't yet know whether cancer cells can develop resistance to fenbendazole specifically, but resistance to microtubule-targeting drugs in general is well-documented. This is one reason why combination therapies are often used—it's harder for cancer cells to develop resistance to multiple drugs simultaneously.

Why Timing Matters: Cell Cycle Synchronization

An interesting aspect of cell cycle-specific drugs like microtubule disruptors is that they only affect cells during certain phases of the cell cycle. Cells in other phases are temporarily resistant.

This creates a challenge: if you give a single dose of a microtubule-disrupting drug, it will only affect cells that happen to be in M phase at that moment. Other cells will be unaffected and will continue dividing.

This is why chemotherapy is typically given in cycles—repeated doses over time ensure that all cancer cells eventually pass through the vulnerable phase while the drug is present.

For fenbendazole, this raises questions about optimal dosing schedules:

- Should it be taken continuously to ensure constant drug presence?
- Should it be taken in cycles to allow normal cells to recover?
- How long does it need to be present to affect all cancer cells?

These questions haven't been answered through formal research, so patients and doctors are left to make educated guesses.

The Immune System and Cancer

Modern cancer treatment increasingly recognizes the crucial role of the immune system. Your immune system can recognize and destroy cancer cells, but cancer cells develop ways to evade immune detection.

Some cancer treatments work by enhancing the immune system's ability to fight cancer:

- Checkpoint inhibitors remove brakes on immune cells
- CAR-T therapy engineers immune cells to target cancer
- Cancer vaccines train the immune system to recognize cancer cells

There's limited research on whether fenbendazole affects the immune system's interaction with cancer. Some studies suggest benzimidazoles may have immunomodulatory effects, but this area needs much more research.

If fenbendazole does enhance immune recognition of cancer cells, it could potentially work synergistically with immunotherapy drugs. But this is speculative at this point.

Metastasis: Cancer's Deadliest Feature

Most cancer deaths aren't caused by the primary tumor—they're caused by metastasis, the spread of cancer to distant organs.

Metastasis is a complex process:

1. Cancer cells break away from the primary tumor

2. They invade surrounding tissue

3. They enter blood vessels or lymphatic vessels

4. They survive in circulation

5. They exit vessels at distant sites

6. They establish new tumors in distant organs

Each step requires specific capabilities. Cancer cells must be able to move, survive outside their original environment, and adapt to new tissue environments.

Microtubules are involved in cell movement, so microtubule-disrupting drugs might theoretically reduce metastasis. Some research in mice suggests fenbendazole may reduce metastatic spread, but this hasn't been confirmed in humans.

Cancer Stem Cells: The Root of Recurrence

A particularly challenging aspect of cancer biology is the existence of cancer stem cells—a small population of cells within tumors that have stem cell-like properties:

- They can self-renew indefinitely
- They can give rise to all other cell types in the tumor
- They're often resistant to conventional treatments
- They may be responsible for cancer recurrence after treatment

If cancer stem cells survive treatment, they can regenerate the entire tumor. This is thought to be one reason why cancers often recur after initially successful treatment.

We don't know whether fenbendazole affects cancer stem cells. If it only affects rapidly dividing cells, it might miss slowly dividing or quiescent cancer stem cells. This is a significant unknown.

Combination Therapy: The Modern Approach

Modern cancer treatment increasingly uses combination approaches:

- Multiple chemotherapy drugs
- Chemotherapy plus targeted therapy
- Chemotherapy plus immunotherapy
- Targeted therapy plus immunotherapy

Combinations work better than single drugs for several reasons:

- They attack cancer through multiple mechanisms
- They reduce the likelihood of resistance
- They may have synergistic effects (the combination is more effective than the sum of individual effects)

If fenbendazole has anti-cancer activity, it would likely be most effective as part of a combination approach rather than as a single agent. Some patients using fenbendazole combine it with:

- Conventional chemotherapy
- Other repurposed drugs

- Supplements thought to enhance its effects
- Immunotherapy

However, combinations also increase the risk of drug interactions and side effects, so they need to be approached carefully.

Personalized Medicine: Not All Cancers Are Equal

Modern oncology increasingly recognizes that cancer treatment needs to be personalized. Two patients with the same cancer type may need different treatments based on:

- The genetic profile of their tumor
- Their overall health and other medical conditions
- Previous treatments and responses
- Personal preferences and values

Genetic testing of tumors can identify specific mutations that predict response to certain drugs. For example:

- EGFR mutations in lung cancer predict response to EGFR inhibitors
- HER2 overexpression in breast cancer predicts response to trastuzumab
- BRCA mutations predict response to PARP inhibitors

We don't yet know whether any genetic markers predict response to fenbendazole. Without this knowledge, it's impossible to predict which patients might benefit most.

Key Takeaways

- Cancer is fundamentally a disease of uncontrolled cell division, making rapidly dividing cells vulnerable to microtubule disruption
- Microtubule-disrupting drugs affect cancer cells more than most normal cells because cancer cells divide more frequently
- Tumor heterogeneity, the microenvironment, and cancer stem cells all complicate treatment
- Drug resistance is a major challenge for all cancer treatments, including microtubule-targeting drugs
- Modern cancer treatment increasingly uses combinations and personalized approaches
- Many aspects of how fenbendazole might work in human cancer remain unknown

PART TWO: THE EVIDENCE—WHAT WE KNOW AND DON'T KNOW

CHAPTER FOUR: LABORATORY RESEARCH

Now that we understand the scientific rationale for fenbendazole's potential anti-cancer effects, let's examine the actual research evidence. We'll start with cell culture studies—research done with cancer cells grown in laboratory dishes.

Cell culture studies are the foundation of cancer drug research. They allow researchers to observe how drugs affect cancer cells in a controlled environment. While they have limitations (cells in a dish don't behave exactly like cells in a living body), they provide crucial initial evidence about whether a drug has anti-cancer activity.

Early Benzimidazole Research

The anti-cancer potential of benzimidazoles wasn't discovered with fenbendazole specifically. Research on this drug class's anti-cancer properties goes back decades.

In the 1970s and 1980s, researchers discovered that mebendazole and other benzimidazoles could inhibit cancer cell growth in culture. These early studies showed that:

- Benzimidazoles could kill various types of cancer cells
- The effect was dose-dependent (higher concentrations killed more cells)
- The mechanism involved microtubule disruption
- Cancer cells were more sensitive than some normal cells

However, this early research didn't lead to clinical development. The effects were modest compared to conventional chemotherapy drugs, and pharmaceutical companies focused on more potent and profitable compounds.

Interest in benzimidazoles for cancer waned until the accidental observations in mouse studies (mentioned in Chapter 2) reignited research in the 2000s.

Fenbendazole-Specific Cell Culture Studies

More recent research has specifically examined fenbendazole's effects on cancer cells. Let's look at some key studies:

Lung Cancer Studies

Several studies have examined fenbendazole's effects on lung cancer cells:

A 2018 study published in *Scientific Reports* examined fenbendazole's effects on non-small cell lung cancer cells. The researchers found that:

- Fenbendazole inhibited cancer cell growth in a dose-dependent manner

- It caused cell cycle arrest in the G2/M phase (preventing cells from completing division)
- It induced apoptosis (programmed cell death)
- It disrupted microtubule formation
- The effects were observed at concentrations that might be achievable in humans

The researchers concluded that fenbendazole showed "**potent anti-cancer effects**" and warranted further investigation.

Another study examined fenbendazole's effects on small cell lung cancer cells (the type Joe Tippens had). The results were similar:

- Significant growth inhibition
- Induction of cell death
- Microtubule disruption
- Enhanced effects when combined with other drugs

Colorectal Cancer Studies

Research on colorectal cancer cells has shown:

- Fenbendazole inhibits growth of multiple colorectal cancer cell lines
- It's effective against cells resistant to conventional chemotherapy
- It may work synergistically with other drugs

- The effects involve both microtubule disruption and metabolic interference

One particularly interesting finding was that fenbendazole affected colorectal cancer cells that had developed resistance to 5-fluorouracil (5-FU), a standard chemotherapy drug. This suggests fenbendazole might work through different mechanisms than conventional drugs and could potentially overcome some forms of drug resistance.

Glioblastoma Studies

Glioblastoma is an aggressive brain cancer with poor prognosis. Research on glioblastoma cells has shown:

- Fenbendazole can cross the blood-brain barrier (at least in laboratory models)
- It inhibits glioblastoma cell growth
- It induces cell death through multiple mechanisms
- It may enhance the effects of radiation therapy

The ability to cross the blood-brain barrier is significant because many drugs can't reach brain tumors effectively. If fenbendazole can reach brain tumors in humans, it might be particularly valuable for brain cancers.

Lymphoma Studies

Research on lymphoma cells has demonstrated:

- Strong growth inhibition
- Induction of apoptosis
- Disruption of cancer cell metabolism
- Potential synergy with conventional lymphoma treatments

Breast Cancer Studies

Studies on breast cancer cells have shown:

- Fenbendazole inhibits growth of various breast cancer subtypes
- It's effective against both hormone-receptor-positive and triple-negative breast cancer cells
- It may enhance the effects of hormonal therapies and chemotherapy
- The effects involve microtubule disruption and metabolic interference

Prostate Cancer Studies

Research on prostate cancer cells has found:

- Growth inhibition at achievable concentrations
- Induction of cell death
- Potential effectiveness against castration-resistant prostate cancer
- Possible synergy with hormonal therapies

Mechanisms Revealed by Cell Culture Studies

Cell culture research has helped elucidate the mechanisms by which fenbendazole affects cancer cells:

Microtubule Disruption

Microscopy studies have directly visualized fenbendazole's effects on microtubules:

- Treated cancer cells show disrupted microtubule networks
- The mitotic spindle (crucial for cell division) fails to form properly
- Cells arrest in mitosis and eventually die

Cell Cycle Effects

Flow cytometry studies (which analyze cell populations) have shown:

- Fenbendazole causes accumulation of cells in G2/M phase
- Cells can't progress through mitosis
- This leads to either cell death or abnormal division resulting in non-viable cells

Apoptosis Induction

Multiple markers of apoptosis have been observed:

- Activation of caspases (enzymes that execute apoptosis)
- DNA fragmentation
- Cell membrane changes characteristic of apoptosis
- Mitochondrial dysfunction

Metabolic Effects

Some studies have examined fenbendazole's effects on cancer cell metabolism:

- Reduced glucose uptake
- Decreased lactate production (a byproduct of glycolysis)

- Mitochondrial dysfunction
- Reduced ATP production (cellular energy)

These metabolic effects suggest fenbendazole may work partly by "starving" cancer cells of energy, complementing its microtubule-disrupting effects.

P53 Activation

Some research has shown that fenbendazole can activate p53, the "guardian of the genome":

- P53 levels increase in treated cells
- P53 target genes are activated
- This contributes to cell cycle arrest and apoptosis

Interestingly, this effect may occur even in cells with mutated p53, suggesting fenbendazole might work through p53-independent pathways as well.

Dose-Response Relationships

A crucial aspect of cell culture research is establishing dose-response relationships—how the effect changes with different drug concentrations.

For fenbendazole, studies have generally shown:

IC50 values: The concentration that inhibits 50% of cell growth (IC50) varies by cancer type but typically ranges from 0.1 to 10 micromolar. For context, this is in a range that might be achievable in human blood with reasonable doses.

Dose-dependent effects: Higher concentrations produce greater growth inhibition and more cell death.

Time-dependent effects: Longer exposure produces greater effects, suggesting sustained drug presence is important.

Selectivity: Cancer cells are generally more sensitive than normal cells, but the selectivity varies. Some studies show 2-5 fold selectivity (cancer cells are 2-5 times more sensitive than normal cells), while others show greater selectivity.

Combination Studies

Many cell culture studies have examined fenbendazole in combination with other treatments:

Chemotherapy Combinations

Fenbendazole has been tested with various chemotherapy drugs:

- With paclitaxel: Synergistic effects in some cancer types
- With cisplatin: Enhanced cell death
- With doxorubicin: Additive or synergistic effects
- With 5-fluorouracil: Overcomes resistance in some cells

"Synergistic" means the combination is more effective than the sum of individual effects—1+1=3, essentially. "Additive" means the effects simply add together—1+1=2.

Radiation Combinations

Some studies have examined fenbendazole with radiation therapy:

- Enhanced radiation-induced cell death
- Possible radiosensitization (making cells more vulnerable to radiation)
- Potential to reduce radiation doses needed

Targeted Therapy Combinations

Research has explored fenbendazole with targeted cancer drugs:

- With EGFR inhibitors in lung cancer
- With hormonal therapies in breast and prostate cancer
- With VEGF inhibitors (anti-angiogenesis drugs)

Results have been mixed, with some combinations showing synergy and others showing only additive effects.

Limitations of Cell Culture Studies

While cell culture studies provide valuable information, they have significant limitations:

Artificial Environment

Cells in culture are in a highly artificial environment:

- They're grown on plastic in nutrient-rich media
- They have unlimited access to oxygen and nutrients
- They lack the three-dimensional structure of real tumors
- They don't interact with immune cells, blood vessels, or other components of the tumor microenvironment

Selection Bias

Cancer cell lines used in research have been selected for their ability to grow in culture. They may not represent the full diversity of cancer cells in actual tumors.

Lack of Pharmacokinetics

In cell culture, researchers can expose cells to specific drug concentrations. In a living body, drug concentrations depend on:

- Absorption from the digestive tract
- Distribution to different tissues
- Metabolism and breakdown
- Excretion

Cell culture studies can't tell us whether achievable drug concentrations in humans will be sufficient for anti-cancer effects.

No Immune System

Cell culture studies can't assess how drugs affect the immune system's interaction with cancer, which is increasingly recognized as crucial for cancer treatment.

Simplified Genetics

Cell lines are genetically simpler than real tumors. They don't capture the genetic heterogeneity and evolution that occurs in actual cancers.

What Cell Culture Studies Tell Us

Despite their limitations, cell culture studies of fenbendazole provide important information:

Proof of Concept: Fenbendazole clearly has anti-cancer activity in laboratory settings. This isn't speculation—it's demonstrated fact.

Mechanism Understanding: We understand how fenbendazole affects cancer cells at the molecular level.

Broad Activity: Fenbendazole shows activity against many cancer types, suggesting broad-spectrum potential.

Achievable Concentrations: The concentrations that show effects in cell culture appear to be in a range that might be achievable in humans.

Combination Potential: Fenbendazole may enhance other treatments, suggesting value in combination approaches.

Safety Margin: Cancer cells appear more sensitive than normal cells, suggesting a therapeutic window exists.

What Cell Culture Studies Don't Tell Us

Equally important is what cell culture studies can't tell us:

Human Efficacy: Will fenbendazole actually work in human cancer patients? Cell culture can't answer this.

Optimal Dosing: What dose should humans take? Cell culture provides hints but not definitive answers.

Safety in Humans: Will the doses needed for anti-cancer effects be safe in humans? Cell culture can't fully address this.

Pharmacokinetics: Will fenbendazole reach tumors in sufficient concentrations in living humans? Unknown.

Long-term Effects: What happens with prolonged use? Cell culture studies are typically short-term.

Patient Selection: Which patients might benefit most? Cell culture can't predict individual responses.

The Translation Challenge

The gap between cell culture success and human clinical success is enormous. Many drugs that work brilliantly in cell culture fail in humans because:

- They can't reach tumors in sufficient concentrations

- They're too toxic at effective doses
- They're metabolized too quickly
- The tumor microenvironment protects cancer cells
- Drug resistance develops
- The cancer biology in humans is more complex than in cell culture

This translation challenge is why we need animal studies and human clinical trials. Cell culture studies are necessary but not sufficient for determining whether a drug will work in patients.

Key Takeaways

- Multiple cell culture studies demonstrate that fenbendazole has anti-cancer activity against various cancer types
- The mechanisms include microtubule disruption, metabolic interference, and induction of cell death
- Effects are dose-dependent and time-dependent
- Fenbendazole may work synergistically with other treatments
- Cell culture studies have significant limitations and can't predict human efficacy
- The concentrations that show effects in cell culture appear potentially achievable in humans, but this needs confirmation

CHAPTER FIVE: ANIMAL STUDIES

Animal studies represent the next step in evaluating potential cancer treatments. They provide crucial information about how drugs work in living organisms, including pharmacokinetics (how the body processes the drug), toxicity, and efficacy against actual tumors.

For fenbendazole, animal research has been particularly important because it was accidental observations in mice that first suggested anti-cancer potential. Let's examine what animal studies have shown.

The Accidental Discovery Revisited

The story of fenbendazole's anti-cancer potential begins with an accident in a research laboratory. Understanding this story helps us appreciate both the promise and the limitations of the evidence.

In the early 2000s, researchers at Johns Hopkins University were conducting experiments with mice that had been genetically engineered to develop cancer. These experiments were designed to test other potential cancer treatments.

The mice were routinely treated with fenbendazole to prevent parasitic infections—standard practice in animal research facilities. But researchers noticed something unexpected: the tumors in these mice weren't growing as expected. In fact, tumor growth was significantly slower than in previous experiments.

After investigation, they realized the difference was the fenbendazole treatment. When they compared mice that received fenbendazole to mice that didn't, the difference was striking: fenbendazole-treated mice had slower tumor growth and longer survival.

This accidental observation led to intentional research. If fenbendazole was affecting tumor growth, it deserved systematic investigation.

Systematic Mouse Studies

Following the accidental discovery, researchers conducted more controlled studies to evaluate fenbendazole's anti-cancer effects in mice.

Lung Cancer Models

Several studies have examined fenbendazole in mouse models of lung cancer:

One study used mice with human lung cancer cells implanted under their skin (xenograft model). The researchers found:

- Fenbendazole treatment significantly reduced tumor growth
- Tumors in treated mice were 40-50% smaller than in untreated mice

- The effect was dose-dependent—higher doses produced greater tumor reduction
- Mice tolerated the treatment well with minimal side effects

Another study used genetically engineered mice that spontaneously develop lung tumors (a more realistic model). Results showed:

- Reduced tumor incidence (fewer mice developed tumors)
- Slower tumor growth in mice that did develop tumors
- Extended survival
- No apparent toxicity at the doses used

Lymphoma Models

Research on lymphoma in mice has shown:

- Significant reduction in tumor burden
- Extended survival
- Enhanced effects when combined with conventional chemotherapy
- Good tolerability

One particularly interesting study examined fenbendazole in mice with drug-resistant lymphoma. The results suggested fenbendazole could overcome some forms of chemotherapy resistance.

Colorectal Cancer Models

Studies in mice with colorectal cancer have demonstrated:

- Reduced tumor growth
- Decreased metastasis to the liver (a common site of colorectal

cancer spread)

- Enhanced effects of conventional chemotherapy
- Minimal toxicity

Glioblastoma Models

Research on brain tumors in mice has shown:

- Fenbendazole can reach brain tumors (crosses the blood-brain barrier)
- Reduced tumor growth
- Extended survival
- Potential synergy with radiation therapy

The ability to reach brain tumors is particularly significant because the blood-brain barrier prevents many drugs from reaching the brain effectively.

Breast Cancer Models

Studies in mice with breast cancer have found:

- Reduced tumor growth across different breast cancer subtypes
- Decreased metastasis to lungs (a common site of breast cancer spread)
- Enhanced effects of hormonal therapies
- Good safety profile

Dosing and Pharmacokinetics in Animals

Animal studies have provided crucial information about fenbendazole's pharmacokinetics—how the body absorbs, distributes, metabolizes, and excretes the drug.

Absorption

Studies have confirmed that fenbendazole is poorly absorbed from the digestive tract in mice, similar to what's known from veterinary use. However:

- Absorption improves when given with fatty foods
- Repeated dosing leads to accumulation in tissues
- Some absorption does occur, enough to reach tumors

Distribution

Research has shown that fenbendazole:

- Distributes to various tissues including tumors
- Crosses the blood-brain barrier to some extent
- Accumulates in liver and fat tissue
- Reaches concentrations in tumors that correlate with anti-cancer effects

Metabolism

Fenbendazole is metabolized in the liver to several compounds:

- Oxfendazole (the primary metabolite, which also has anti-cancer activity)
- Fenbendazole sulfone

- Other minor metabolites

The fact that metabolites also have activity means the drug's effects may be prolonged beyond the presence of the parent compound.

Excretion

Fenbendazole and its metabolites are excreted primarily in feces, with some urinary excretion. The half-life in mice is approximately 10-15 hours, meaning the drug is cleared relatively quickly.

Dose Translation

Translating doses from mice to humans is complex. Mice metabolize drugs faster than humans due to their higher metabolic rate and different body surface area to weight ratio.

The doses used in mouse studies typically range from 50-200 mg/kg body weight. Using standard conversion factors, this translates to approximately 4-16 mg/kg in humans, or roughly 280-1,120mg for a 70 kg (154 lb) adult. However, this is a rough estimate, and the actual effective dose in humans remains unknown.

It's worth noting that many patients who use fenbendazole take doses in the range of 200-300 mg per day (approximately 3-4 mg/kg for a 70 kg person), which is at the lower end of the translated range from mouse studies. Whether this is sufficient to achieve anti-cancer effects in humans is uncertain.

Toxicity and Safety in Animals

One of the most encouraging findings from animal studies is that fenbendazole appears to be well-tolerated even at doses that show anti-cancer effects.

Acute Toxicity

Studies examining single high doses of fenbendazole in mice and rats have found:

- The LD50 (dose that kills 50% of animals) is very high—greater than 10,000 mg/kg in mice
- This means fenbendazole has a very wide safety margin
- Acute toxicity is rare even at doses far exceeding those used for anti-cancer effects

Chronic Toxicity

More relevant to cancer treatment are studies of repeated dosing over weeks or months:

- Mice treated with fenbendazole daily for several weeks show minimal toxicity
- Weight loss is minimal or absent at anti-cancer doses
- Liver enzyme elevations are mild and reversible
- Blood cell counts remain largely normal
- Organ damage is not observed at therapeutic doses

Comparison to Chemotherapy

When compared to conventional chemotherapy drugs in the same mouse models:

- Fenbendazole causes significantly less weight loss
- It produces less bone marrow suppression (fewer effects on blood cells)
- It causes less gastrointestinal toxicity

- Mice appear healthier and more active during treatment

This favorable toxicity profile is one reason fenbendazole has attracted interest as a potential cancer treatment.

Species Differences

It's important to note that toxicity can vary between species. What's safe in mice may not be equally safe in humans, and vice versa. However, fenbendazole's long history of safe use in multiple animal species (dogs, cats, horses, cattle, etc.) provides reassurance about its general safety profile.

Safety Margins and Therapeutic Windows

A crucial concept in drug development is the "therapeutic window"—the range between doses that are effective and doses that are toxic.

For fenbendazole in mice:

- Effective anti-cancer doses: 50-200 mg/kg
- Toxic doses: >10,000 mg/kg
- Therapeutic window: approximately 50-200 fold

This wide therapeutic window is encouraging. For comparison, many chemotherapy drugs have therapeutic windows of only 2-5 fold, meaning the difference between an effective dose and a toxic dose is very small.

However, we must be cautious about assuming this wide therapeutic window translates to humans. Humans may metabolize fenbendazole differently, may be more or less sensitive to its effects, and may experience toxicities that don't occur in mice.

Combination Toxicity

Several animal studies have examined fenbendazole in combination with other cancer treatments:

With Chemotherapy

When combined with conventional chemotherapy drugs:

- Toxicity is generally not increased beyond what's expected from chemotherapy alone
- In some cases, fenbendazole may actually reduce chemotherapy side effects
- No unexpected or synergistic toxicities have been observed

With Radiation

Studies combining fenbendazole with radiation therapy have found:

- No increase in radiation-induced toxicity
- Possible protective effects on normal tissues
- Enhanced tumor response without increased side effects

With Targeted Therapies

Limited research on combinations with targeted cancer drugs suggests:

- Generally well-tolerated combinations
- No major drug-drug interactions observed
- Potential for enhanced efficacy without increased toxicity

These findings suggest that fenbendazole might be safely combined with conventional treatments, though human data is needed to confirm this.

Long-Term Effects

Some animal studies have examined longer-term treatment with fenbendazole:

- Mice treated for several months show no cumulative toxicity
- Organ function remains normal
- No evidence of carcinogenicity (cancer-causing effects)
- Fertility and reproduction appear unaffected

However, these studies are still relatively short compared to human lifespans, and very long-term effects remain unknown.

Limitations of Animal Toxicity Studies

While animal studies provide valuable safety information, they have limitations:

Species Differences

Humans may respond differently than mice to fenbendazole. We may:

- Metabolize it differently
- Be more or less sensitive to its effects
- Experience toxicities that don't occur in mice
- Require different doses to achieve the same effects

Study Duration

Most animal studies last weeks to months, not years. Long-term effects in humans using fenbendazole for extended periods are unknown.

Genetic Diversity

Laboratory mice are genetically uniform, while humans are genetically diverse. Some people may be more susceptible to side effects due to genetic variations in drug metabolism.

Concurrent Medications

Humans, especially cancer patients, often take multiple medications. Drug interactions that don't occur in mice might occur in humans taking other drugs.

Underlying Health Conditions

Cancer patients often have compromised health, which may make them more vulnerable to side effects than healthy mice.

What Animal Studies Tell Us

Animal studies of fenbendazole provide several important pieces of information:

1. **Proof of Concept**: Fenbendazole can slow tumor growth and extend survival in multiple cancer models

2. **Mechanism Confirmation**: The anti-cancer effects involve microtubule disruption, metabolic interference, and apoptosis induction

3. **Dose-Response**: Higher doses produce greater effects, up to a point

4. **Safety Profile**: Fenbendazole appears well-tolerated at doses

that show anti-cancer activity

5. **Combination Potential**: It can be safely combined with conventional treatments in mice

6. **Broad Activity**: It shows effects against multiple cancer types

What Animal Studies Don't Tell Us

Equally important is what animal studies cannot tell us:

1. **Human Efficacy**: Whether fenbendazole will work in human cancer patients

2. **Optimal Dosing**: What dose is most effective in humans

3. **Long-Term Safety**: Effects of years of use in humans

4. **Patient Selection**: Which patients might benefit most

5. **Combination Effects**: How it interacts with the full range of human cancer treatments

6. **Quality of Life**: How it affects patients' day-to-day experience

The Translation Gap

The gap between promising animal studies and human benefit is substantial. History is full of treatments that worked brilliantly in mice but failed in humans:

- Different tumor biology between species
- Different immune systems
- Different drug metabolism
- Different tumor microenvironments
- Different genetic complexity

This is why clinical trials in humans are essential. No amount of animal research can substitute for carefully conducted human studies.

Key Takeaways

- Animal studies demonstrate that fenbendazole has anti-cancer activity in multiple mouse models of cancer
- It slows tumor growth, reduces tumor size, and extends survival in mice
- The doses that show anti-cancer effects in mice translate to approximately 280-1,120 mg daily for a 70 kg human, though this is uncertain
- Fenbendazole appears well-tolerated in animals with minimal toxicity at therapeutic doses
- It has a wide therapeutic window (large gap between effective and toxic doses)
- It can be safely combined with conventional treatments in animal models

- However, animal studies cannot predict whether fenbendazole will work in human cancer patients
- Clinical trials in humans are needed to determine efficacy, optimal dosing, and safety in people
- The translation from animal success to human benefit is uncertain and requires formal clinical research

CHAPTER SIX: HUMAN EVIDENCE

This is where the story of fenbendazole and cancer becomes both more interesting and more complicated. We have compelling laboratory research and promising animal studies. But what about evidence in actual human cancer patients?

The short answer is: we have very limited formal evidence, but we have many patient reports and anecdotal accounts. Understanding the difference between these types of evidence—and what each can and cannot tell us—is crucial for making informed decisions.

The Current State of Human Evidence

Let's be direct: as of this writing, there are no published, peer-reviewed clinical trials of fenbendazole as a cancer treatment in humans.[2026] None.

This is a critical fact that must be understood clearly. When oncologists say "there's no evidence that fenbendazole works for cancer," this is what they mean: there are no formal clinical trials demonstrating efficacy in human patients.

What we do have is:

- One famous case report (Joe Tippens)
- Numerous anecdotal reports from patients
- Crowdsourced data from online communities
- Informal observations from some physicians
- Case series being compiled by interested researchers

This type of evidence is fundamentally different from clinical trial data. It can suggest possibilities and generate hypotheses, but it cannot prove that a treatment works.

Why Clinical Trials Haven't Happened

Given the promising laboratory and animal research, why hasn't anyone conducted a proper clinical trial of fenbendazole for cancer? The reasons are complex and reveal much about how medical research is funded and conducted.

Patent and Profit Issues

Fenbendazole is a generic drug that's been off-patent for decades. This means:

- Any pharmaceutical company can manufacture it
- No company can have exclusive rights to sell it
- There's no way to recoup the $100+ million cost of clinical

trials

- No financial incentive exists for companies to fund research

This is the fundamental problem with repurposed drugs. Even if they work, the economics of drug development don't support the research needed to prove it.

Regulatory Barriers

To conduct a clinical trial, researchers need:

- Approval from institutional review boards (IRBs)
- An Investigational New Drug (IND) application with the FDA
- Good Manufacturing Practice (GMP) grade drug supply
- Liability insurance
- Regulatory expertise

These requirements are designed to protect patients, but they also create barriers to studying repurposed drugs. Fenbendazole is approved for veterinary use, not human use, which complicates regulatory approval.

Academic Incentives

Academic researchers typically focus on:

- Novel mechanisms and new discoveries
- Patentable innovations
- Fundable research (grants from NIH, foundations, etc.)
- Publishable results in high-impact journals

Studying a generic veterinary drug doesn't align well with these incentives. It's not novel, it's not patentable, and it's hard to get funded.

Risk Aversion

Cancer researchers and oncologists are understandably cautious about:

- Recommending unproven treatments
- Being associated with "alternative" medicine
- Potential harm to patients
- Damage to professional reputation

This caution is appropriate, but it can also slow investigation of promising but unconventional approaches.

The Catch-22

This creates a catch-22 situation:

- Without clinical trials, there's no proof fenbendazole works
- Without proof, doctors won't recommend it
- Without doctor support, it's hard to conduct trials
- Without financial incentive, no one will fund trials
- Without trials, there's no proof...

This cycle is difficult to break, and it affects many potentially useful repurposed drugs, not just fenbendazole.

The Joe Tippens Case: The Story That Started It All

Joe Tippens' story is the reason most people have heard about fenbendazole and cancer. His case is remarkable, but it's also important to understand what it does and doesn't prove.

The Basic Story

In 2016, Joe Tippens was diagnosed with small cell lung cancer that had metastasized extensively. His doctors gave him a grim prognosis—months to live. He underwent conventional treatment including chemotherapy.

During his treatment, a veterinarian friend told him about a scientist who had cured cancer in mice using fenbendazole. Facing a terminal diagnosis, Tippens decided to try it. He took fenbendazole (222 mg daily) along with several supplements:

- Vitamin E
- Curcumin
- CBD oil

He continued his conventional cancer treatment while adding the fenbendazole protocol.

The Outcome

After several months, scans showed that Tippens' cancer had disappeared. His oncologists were surprised—small cell lung cancer rarely responds this well to treatment, especially when it has metastasized extensively.

Tippens has remained cancer-free for years. He attributes his recovery to fenbendazole and has shared his story widely through his blog, social media, and interviews.

Tippens was also the participant in a clinical trial at MD Anderson involving the immunotherapy drug Keytruda. (Pembrolizumab)

While on the Keytruda trial, he[Tippens] also began self-administering fenbendazole with other supplements. His subsequent remission was widely publicized as a "fenbendazole miracle," but medical experts suggest his positive outcome was likely due to the immunotherapy trial rather than the unproven animal drug. MD Anderson does not support the use of fenbendazole for human cancer treatment. While a former patient's story involved the drug, his treatment and recovery likely came from an official clinical trial conducted at MD Anderson using a different immunotherapy medication.

What This Case Tells Us

Joe Tippens' case is remarkable and deserves attention. It suggests that something unusual happened. Possible explanations include:

1. **Fenbendazole worked**: The drug had anti-cancer effects in Tippens
2. **Conventional treatment worked**: His chemotherapy was more effective than expected
3. **Combination effect**: Fenbendazole enhanced his chemotherapy
4. **Supplements helped**: The vitamins and supplements he took had effects
5. **Spontaneous remission**: His cancer regressed on its own (rare but documented)
6. **Immune response**: His immune system mounted an unusually effective response
7. **Combination of factors**: Multiple factors worked together

We cannot know which explanation is correct based on a single case.

What This Case Doesn't Tell Us

As compelling as Tippens' story is, a single case cannot prove that fenbendazole works for cancer. Here's why:

No Control Group: We don't know what would have happened if Tippens had not taken fenbendazole. Maybe his chemotherapy alone would have worked just as well.

Multiple Interventions: Tippens took fenbendazole plus supplements plus chemotherapy. We can't isolate which factor (or combination) was responsible for his recovery.

Sample Size of One: One person's experience, no matter how dramatic, cannot establish that a treatment works. Individual responses to cancer treatment vary enormously.

Publication Bias: We hear about dramatic successes like Tippens' story. We don't hear about the patients who tried fenbendazole and didn't respond. This creates a distorted picture.

Confirmation Bias: Once Tippens attributed his recovery to fenbendazole, he naturally focused on evidence supporting this belief and may have discounted alternative explanations.

Rare but Possible: Unexpected remissions do occur with conventional treatment alone, especially with modern chemotherapy regimens. Tippens' response, while unusual, is not impossible without fenbendazole.

Other Patient Reports: The Crowdsourced Evidence

Following Tippens' story, thousands of cancer patients have tried fenbendazole. Many have shared their experiences online, creating a crowdsourced database of patient reports.

Where to Find Reports

Patient experiences are shared in various places:

- Facebook groups dedicated to fenbendazole and cancer
- Online forums and message boards
- The Telegram channel mentioned earlier [https://t.me/fen bendazol]
- Personal blogs and websites
- YouTube videos and testimonials

These communities have become repositories of patient experiences, dosing information, and practical advice.

Types of Reports

The reports vary widely:

Positive Reports: Some patients report:

- Tumor shrinkage on scans
- Improved symptoms
- Stable disease when progression was expected
- Better tolerance of conventional treatment
- Improved quality of life

Neutral Reports: Many patients report:

- No obvious change in their cancer
- Continued disease progression despite fenbendazole
- Uncertain whether it's helping

Negative Reports: Some patients report:

- Side effects from fenbendazole

- Continued cancer progression
- Disappointment that it didn't work
- Regret about trying it

The Selection Bias Problem

Here's a critical issue: positive reports are much more likely to be shared than negative ones. This creates selection bias:

- Patients whose cancer responds are excited to share their success
- Patients whose cancer progresses may be too ill to post updates
- Patients who see no benefit may quietly stop taking it
- Patients who die are obviously unable to report their experience

This means the online reports we see are not representative of all patients who try fenbendazole. They're skewed toward positive outcomes.

The Plural of Anecdote Is Not Data

There's a saying in medicine: "The plural of anecdote is not data." Even hundreds of patient reports cannot substitute for a properly conducted clinical trial. Here's why:

No Standardization: Patients take different doses, different formulations, different combinations of supplements, and different conventional treatments. There's no way to know what's causing any observed effects.

No Verification: Patient reports are self-reported and unverified. We don't know if:

- The cancer diagnosis was accurate
- The scans were interpreted correctly
- Other treatments were being used
- The timeline is accurate

No Follow-Up: Many reports are snapshots in time. We don't know what happened to these patients long-term.

Confounding Factors: Cancer patients are typically receiving multiple treatments. Any observed effects could be due to:

- Conventional chemotherapy
- Radiation therapy
- Immunotherapy
- Other supplements or medications
- Dietary changes
- Natural disease fluctuation

Reporting Bias: Patients who believe fenbendazole is working may interpret stable disease as success, while patients not taking it might view the same outcome as failure.

What Doctors Are Observing

Some oncologists have patients who use fenbendazole, either with or without their knowledge. What are doctors seeing?

Informal Observations

A few oncologists have informally noted:

- Some patients taking fenbendazole have had good responses to treatment
- It's impossible to know if fenbendazole contributed or if conventional treatment was responsible
- Most patients taking fenbendazole also progress, just like patients not taking it
- Side effects appear minimal in most cases

The Attribution Problem

When a patient taking both chemotherapy and fenbendazole responds well, doctors face an attribution problem:

- The chemotherapy is a proven treatment
- Fenbendazole is unproven
- The logical conclusion is that chemotherapy worked
- But we can't rule out that fenbendazole helped

This uncertainty cuts both ways. We can't prove fenbendazole helped, but we also can't prove it didn't.

Physician Reluctance

Most oncologists are reluctant to recommend fenbendazole because:

- There's no clinical trial evidence
- They could face liability if something goes wrong
- It might give patients false hope
- It might delay or interfere with proven treatments

- Professional guidelines don't support its use

However, some oncologists take a more permissive approach:

- They don't recommend it, but they don't forbid it
- They monitor patients who choose to use it
- They're open to discussing it as part of shared decision-making
- They're interested in observing outcomes

The Need for Systematic Data Collection

Several physicians and researchers have recognized that patient experiences, while not proof, are valuable information. Some efforts are underway to:

- Systematically collect patient reports
- Document outcomes more carefully
- Track side effects and safety issues
- Identify patterns that might guide future research

These efforts are preliminary but represent a step toward more rigorous evidence.

Case Series and Observational Data

A "case series" is a step up from individual anecdotes. It involves systematically documenting multiple cases using standardized methods. While not as rigorous as a clinical trial, a well-done case series can provide useful information.

Attempts at Case Series

Some researchers and physicians have attempted to compile case series of patients using fenbendazole:

- Collecting medical records
- Documenting cancer types and stages
- Recording treatment protocols
- Following outcomes over time
- Analyzing patterns

However, these efforts face challenges:

- Patients are geographically dispersed
- Medical records are often incomplete
- Patients use varying protocols
- Follow-up is difficult
- Funding is limited

What Case Series Could Tell Us

A well-conducted case series could provide:

- Better estimates of response rates
- Information about which cancer types might respond
- Data on safety and side effects
- Insights into optimal dosing
- Hypotheses for future clinical trials

However, even a good case series cannot prove causation. It can only describe what happened to patients who used fenbendazole, not whether fenbendazole caused any observed effects.

The Problem with Anecdotal Evidence

It's worth exploring in detail why anecdotal evidence, no matter how compelling, cannot prove that a treatment works.

Selection Bias

We've mentioned this, but it's worth emphasizing. The cases we hear about are not representative:

- Dramatic successes get shared widely
- Modest benefits may not be reported
- Failures are often silent
- Deaths end the possibility of reporting

This creates a distorted picture where fenbendazole appears more effective than it actually is.

Confirmation Bias

Once someone believes fenbendazole is working, they interpret events through that lens:

- Stable disease becomes "fenbendazole is working"
- Slow progression becomes "it's slowing the cancer"
- Side effects from chemotherapy become "detox reactions"
- Any improvement is attributed to fenbendazole

This isn't dishonesty—it's human nature. We all interpret ambiguous information in ways that confirm our existing beliefs.

The Post Hoc Fallacy

"Post hoc ergo propter hoc" means "after this, therefore because of this." It's a logical fallacy:

- Patient takes fenbendazole
- Patient's cancer improves
- Therefore, fenbendazole caused the improvement

This logic is flawed because:

- The improvement might have happened anyway
- Other treatments might be responsible
- Natural disease fluctuation might explain it
- Spontaneous remission, while rare, does occur

Regression to the Mean

Cancer doesn't progress in a straight line. It fluctuates:

- Tumors may grow, then stabilize, then grow again
- Symptoms may worsen, then improve, then worsen
- Scans may show progression, then stability, then progression

Patients often start new treatments when their cancer is at its worst. Natural fluctuation means some improvement is likely regardless of treatment. This improvement gets attributed to the new treatment.

The Placebo Effect

The placebo effect is real and powerful, especially for subjective outcomes like:

- Pain levels
- Energy and fatigue
- Mood and anxiety
- Quality of life

Patients who believe fenbendazole is helping may genuinely feel better, even if the drug has no direct anti-cancer effect. This doesn't mean they're imagining it—placebo effects involve real physiological changes.

However, placebo effects are less likely to affect objective outcomes like tumor size on scans.

Distinguishing Correlation from Causation

The fundamental challenge with anecdotal evidence is distinguishing correlation (two things happening together) from causation (one thing causing another).

Correlation Examples

Consider these scenarios:

Scenario 1: A patient takes fenbendazole while receiving chemotherapy. The cancer responds. Did fenbendazole help, or did chemotherapy work as intended?

Scenario 2: A patient takes fenbendazole after completing chemotherapy. The cancer remains stable. Is this due to fenbendazole, or is it the lasting effect of chemotherapy?

Scenario 3: A patient takes fenbendazole and multiple supplements. The cancer shrinks. Which intervention was responsible?

In each case, we observe correlation (fenbendazole use and cancer response), but we cannot establish causation.

What Would Prove Causation?

To prove that fenbendazole causes cancer regression, we would need:

1. **Temporal relationship**: Fenbendazole use precedes cancer response
2. **Dose-response**: Higher doses produce greater effects
3. **Consistency**: The effect is observed repeatedly across multiple patients
4. **Biological plausibility**: A mechanism explains how fenbendazole could work
5. **Specificity**: The effect is specific to fenbendazole, not other factors
6. **Experimental evidence**: Controlled studies show the effect

We have #1 (temporal relationship) and #4 (biological plausibility) from laboratory research. We lack #2, #3, #5, and #6 in humans.

What Would Real Evidence Look Like?

To truly know whether fenbendazole works for cancer, we need properly conducted clinical trials. What would these look like?

Phase I Trial: Safety and Dosing

The first step would be a Phase I trial to determine:

- What dose is safe in humans?
- What side effects occur?

- How is the drug metabolized?
- What blood levels are achieved?
- What is the maximum tolerated dose?

This would involve a small number of patients (20-40) with advanced cancer. The goal is safety, not efficacy.

Phase II Trial: Preliminary Efficacy

If Phase I shows fenbendazole is safe, Phase II would examine:

- Does it show any anti-cancer activity?
- What cancer types respond?
- What is the response rate?
- What is the optimal dose?

This would involve 40-100 patients with specific cancer types. The goal is to see if there's enough activity to justify larger trials.

Phase III Trial: Definitive Efficacy

If Phase II shows promise, Phase III would definitively test:

- Does fenbendazole improve survival compared to standard treatment?
- Does it improve quality of life?
- What are the long-term side effects?
- Is it cost-effective?

This would involve hundreds or thousands of patients randomly assigned to receive fenbendazole or not. This is the gold standard for proving a treatment works.

Why Randomization Matters

The key feature of Phase III trials is randomization—patients are randomly assigned to treatment groups. This ensures:

- Groups are comparable at the start
- Differences in outcomes are due to treatment, not other factors
- Bias is minimized
- Results are reliable

Without randomization, we can't rule out that observed differences are due to:

- Patient selection (healthier patients choosing fenbendazole)
- Other treatments
- Natural disease variation
- Reporting bias

The Control Group Problem

A major challenge for a fenbendazole trial is the control group. What would patients in the control group receive?

- **Placebo**: Ethically problematic if patients have treatable cancer
- **Standard treatment**: Both groups would receive this, with fenbendazole added to one group
- **Best supportive care**: Only appropriate for patients with no other options

Most likely, a trial would add fenbendazole to standard treatment and compare outcomes to standard treatment alone.

Endpoints and Outcomes

Clinical trials measure specific endpoints:

- **Overall survival**: How long patients live
- **Progression-free survival**: How long until cancer worsens
- **Response rate**: Percentage of patients whose tumors shrink
- **Quality of life**: Patient-reported outcomes
- **Toxicity**: Side effects and safety

These objective measures are more reliable than patient testimonials.

The Time and Cost

A complete clinical trial program would take:

- 5-10 years to complete all phases
- $50-100 million in funding
- Hundreds of patients willing to participate
- Regulatory approval and oversight
- Expert investigators and research staff

This is why clinical trials are so rare for repurposed drugs—the investment is enormous and the financial return is minimal.

Alternative Research Models

Given the barriers to traditional clinical trials, some researchers are exploring alternative models:

Pragmatic Trials

These trials are designed to be simpler and cheaper:

- Less restrictive eligibility criteria
- Fewer study visits and tests
- Use of existing medical records
- Comparison to real-world standard care

Pragmatic trials sacrifice some rigor for feasibility and cost-effectiveness.

Registry Studies

These involve systematically tracking patients who choose to use fenbendazole:

- Collecting baseline data
- Following outcomes over time
- Comparing to matched controls
- Analyzing patterns

While not as rigorous as randomized trials, registries can provide useful real-world data.

N-of-1 Trials

These are trials in individual patients:

- Patient alternates between fenbendazole and no fenbendazole
- Outcomes are tracked carefully

- Patient serves as their own control

Multiple N-of-1 trials can be combined to draw conclusions.

Crowdsourced Data

Some researchers are exploring ways to harness patient-reported data:

- Online platforms for data collection
- Standardized reporting forms
- Statistical methods to account for bias
- Large numbers to overcome individual variation

This approach is experimental but could provide insights.

The Ethical Dilemma

The lack of clinical trial evidence creates an ethical dilemma:

For Patients:

- Should they try an unproven treatment?
- How do they weigh potential benefits against unknown risks?
- Is it ethical to use themselves as experimental subjects?

For Doctors:

- Should they support patients who want to try fenbendazole?
- Is it ethical to recommend an unproven treatment?
- How do they balance patient autonomy with professional responsibility?

For Researchers:

- Should they prioritize studying fenbendazole despite funding challenges?
- Is it ethical to conduct trials when financial incentives are lacking?
- How do they balance scientific rigor with patient urgency?

For Society:

- Should we fund research on repurposed drugs?
- How do we balance innovation with evidence standards?
- What responsibility do we have to patients with limited options?

These questions don't have easy answers, but they're worth grappling with.

Key Takeaways

- There are no published clinical trials of fenbendazole for cancer in humans
- The lack of trials is due to financial, regulatory, and practical barriers, not lack of scientific interest
- Joe Tippens' case is remarkable but cannot prove fenbendazole works—it's a single case with multiple confounding factors
- Numerous patient reports exist, but they suffer from selec-

tion bias, reporting bias, and lack of verification

- Anecdotal evidence, no matter how abundant, cannot establish causation or prove efficacy
- Doctors who observe patients using fenbendazole cannot determine whether it's helping due to confounding factors
- Properly conducted clinical trials would require randomization, control groups, objective endpoints, and years of research
- Alternative research models (pragmatic trials, registries, crowdsourced data) may provide some insights but cannot replace formal trials
- The lack of evidence creates ethical dilemmas for patients, doctors, researchers, and society
- Patients considering fenbendazole must understand they are essentially participating in an uncontrolled experiment on themselves
- The gap between promising laboratory research and proven human benefit remains large and can only be bridged by formal clinical research

PART THREE: PRACTICAL GUIDANCE FOR PATIENTS AND FAMILIES

If you've read this far, you understand both the promise and the limitations of fenbendazole as a potential cancer treatment. You know the laboratory research is intriguing, the animal studies are encouraging, but the human evidence is limited to anecdotal reports and case studies.

Now comes the practical question: What do you actually do with this information?

This section is designed to help you navigate the real-world decisions you face. Whether you're considering fenbendazole for yourself or a loved one, or simply want to understand it better, these chapters provide practical guidance on:

- How to evaluate the flood of information you'll encounter online
- How to have productive conversations with your healthcare team
- The practical aspects of sourcing, dosing, and using fenbendazole
- How to monitor for effects and side effects
- Safety considerations and potential interactions
- How to integrate fenbendazole with conventional treatment
- Legal and regulatory considerations

Throughout this section, we'll be honest about what's known and what isn't. We'll provide practical guidance while acknowledging the uncertainties. And we'll emphasize repeatedly that these decisions should be made in consultation with qualified healthcare providers who know your specific situation.

Let's begin with perhaps the most important skill for any patient in the internet age: how to critically evaluate health information.

CHAPTER SEVEN: EVALUATING INFORMATION AND RESEARCH

When you start researching fenbendazole and cancer, you'll be overwhelmed by information. Blog posts, YouTube videos, Facebook groups, scientific papers, news articles, testimonials, and more. Some of this information is reliable and helpful. Much of it is not.

Learning to distinguish good information from bad is perhaps the most important skill you can develop as a patient or caregiver. This chapter will teach you how to think critically about health information, evaluate sources, understand research, and avoid common pitfalls.

The Information Landscape: What You'll Encounter

Let's start by mapping the types of information you'll find about fenbendazole and cancer:

Patient Testimonials and Anecdotes

These are personal stories from people who have used fenbendazole. You'll find them on:

- Facebook groups and online forums
- Personal blogs and websites
- YouTube videos
- The Telegram channel and similar platforms

Strengths: Provide real-world experiences, practical tips, emotional support**Weaknesses**: Subject to bias, unverified, lack controls, can't establish causation

News Articles and Media Coverage

Mainstream and alternative media have covered the fenbendazole story. These articles range from:

- Balanced reporting on the phenomenon
- Sensationalized "miracle cure" stories
- Skeptical debunking pieces

Strengths: May introduce you to the topic, sometimes cite experts**Weaknesses**: Often oversimplified, may be sensationalized, rarely provide full context

Health Blogs and Alternative Medicine Websites

Many websites promote fenbendazole and other alternative cancer treatments:

- Natural health blogs
- Alternative medicine practitioners' sites
- Supplement sellers' websites

Strengths: May compile information in one place, sometimes cite research**Weaknesses**: Often have financial conflicts of interest, may cherry-pick evidence, frequently overstate benefits

Scientific Research Papers

These are the primary research studies published in scientific journals:

- Cell culture studies
- Animal studies
- Case reports
- Review articles

Strengths: Peer-reviewed, detailed methods, primary source of evidence**Weaknesses**: Technical language, may be behind paywalls, require expertise to interpret

Medical and Scientific Reviews

Some doctors and scientists have written about fenbendazole:

- Medical blog posts
- Scientific commentary
- Expert opinions

Strengths: Expert perspective, balanced analysis, context**Weaknesses**: Rare (few experts have written about this), may be overly cautious

Social Media Discussions

Twitter, Reddit, Facebook, and other platforms host discussions:

- Patient communities
- Scientific discussions
- Debates between proponents and skeptics

Strengths: Real-time information, diverse perspectives, community support**Weaknesses**: Unverified information, echo chambers, emotional rather than evidence-based

Critical Thinking Fundamentals

Before we dive into specific evaluation strategies, let's establish some fundamental principles of critical thinking about health information.

Principle 1: Extraordinary Claims Require Extraordinary Evidence

When you see claims like "fenbendazole cures cancer" or "this simple drug that doctors don't want you to know about," your skepticism should increase. Extraordinary claims need strong evidence to support them.

Ask yourself:

- Is this claim too good to be true?
- What level of evidence would be needed to support this claim?
- Does the available evidence meet that standard?

Principle 2: Correlation Does Not Equal Causation

Just because two things happen together doesn't mean one caused the other. This is the fundamental problem with anecdotal reports:

- Patient takes fenbendazole
- Patient's cancer improves
- Therefore, fenbendazole caused the improvement (maybe, maybe not)

Always ask:

- What else could explain this outcome?
- How can we rule out alternative explanations?
- Is there a plausible mechanism?

Principle 3: Anecdotes Are Not Data

Personal stories are compelling, but they're not scientific evidence. A thousand anecdotes don't equal one well-designed study.

Remember:

- Anecdotes suffer from selection bias (we hear about successes, not failures)
- They lack controls (we don't know what would have happened without the intervention)
- They can't establish causation
- They're subject to reporting bias and memory errors

Principle 4: Consider the Source

Who is providing this information, and what are their motivations? Ask:

- What are their credentials and expertise?

- Do they have financial conflicts of interest?
- Are they selling something?
- What is their track record for accuracy?

Principle 5: Look for Consensus, Not Outliers

One study or one expert saying something different from the mainstream doesn't make them right. Scientific consensus develops over time through replication and peer review.

Be wary of:

- "Maverick" doctors or scientists claiming everyone else is wrong
- Single studies that contradict a body of evidence
- Claims that "they" don't want you to know

Principle 6: Understand Your Own Biases

We all have biases that affect how we interpret information:

- **Confirmation bias**: We seek out and believe information that confirms what we already think
- **Motivated reasoning**: We evaluate evidence differently depending on whether we want it to be true
- **Availability bias**: We overweight vivid, memorable examples
- **Optimism bias**: We believe good outcomes are more likely for us than statistics suggest

Being aware of these biases doesn't eliminate them, but it helps you compensate for them.

Evaluating Online Health Information

Now let's get practical. When you encounter health information online, here's how to evaluate it:

Step 1: Check the Source

Look at who published the information:

Reliable Sources (generally trustworthy):

- Peer-reviewed scientific journals
- Major medical institutions (Mayo Clinic, Cleveland Clinic, etc.)
- Government health agencies (NIH, FDA, CDC)
- Professional medical organizations
- Academic medical centers

Moderately Reliable Sources (use with caution):

- Mainstream news outlets with science reporters
- Health-focused news sites (WebMD, Healthline, etc.)
- Medical blogs by credentialed professionals
- Patient advocacy organizations

Unreliable Sources (be very skeptical):

- Sites selling products
- Anonymous blogs or forums
- Social media posts without sources

- Sites with sensationalized headlines
- Alternative medicine sites making extreme claims

Step 2: Look for Citations and References

Good health information cites its sources. Look for:

- Links to scientific studies
- References to specific research
- Quotes from named experts
- Publication dates

Red flags:

- No sources cited
- Vague references ("studies show...")
- Cherry-picked citations that ignore contradictory evidence
- Outdated information

Step 3: Check the Date

Medical information changes rapidly. Information from 2015 may be outdated by 2024. Always check:

- When was this published?
- Has newer research emerged?
- Are the citations recent?

Step 4: Evaluate the Tone and Language

How information is presented tells you a lot:

Good signs:

- Balanced presentation of benefits and risks
- Acknowledgment of uncertainty
- Nuanced language ("may," "suggests," "preliminary")
- Discussion of limitations

Red flags:

- Absolute claims ("cures," "miracle," "guaranteed")
- Emotional manipulation
- Conspiracy theories
- Attacks on conventional medicine
- Pressure to act quickly

Step 5: Look for Financial Conflicts

Is someone trying to sell you something?

- Does the site sell fenbendazole or related products?
- Are there affiliate links?
- Is this sponsored content?
- Does the author have financial ties to companies?

Financial conflicts don't automatically invalidate information, but they should increase your skepticism.

Step 6: Cross-Reference Information

Don't rely on a single source. Check whether:

- Multiple independent sources report the same information

- Reputable sources confirm the claims
- There's scientific consensus or controversy

If only one source makes a claim, be very skeptical.

Understanding Scientific Papers

Scientific research papers are the gold standard for medical evidence, but they're written for other scientists, not the general public. Here's how to approach them:

Types of Scientific Papers

Original Research Articles: Report new experimental findings

- Most valuable for understanding what research actually shows
- Include methods, results, and discussion sections
- Peer-reviewed before publication

Review Articles: Summarize existing research on a topic

- Good for getting an overview
- Should cite many original studies
- Can be biased by author's perspective

Case Reports: Describe individual patient experiences

- Interesting but limited evidence value
- Can't establish causation
- Useful for generating hypotheses

Meta-Analyses: Statistically combine results from multiple studies

- Highest level of evidence when done well
- Only as good as the studies included
- Can be affected by publication bias

Where to Find Scientific Papers

PubMed (pubmed.ncbi.nlm.nih.gov)

- Free database of biomedical literature
- Maintained by the National Library of Medicine
- Includes abstracts (summaries) of most papers
- Some full-text articles available free

Google Scholar (scholar.google.com)

- Searches academic literature across disciplines
- Often finds free versions of papers
- Less comprehensive than PubMed for medical research

Journal Websites

- Many journals make some articles free
- Others require subscriptions or payment
- Some authors post free versions on their websites

How to Use PubMed

Let's walk through a PubMed search for fenbendazole and cancer:

1. Go to pubmed.ncbi.nlm.nih.gov

2. Enter search terms: "fenbendazole cancer"

3. Review the results list

4. Click on titles that seem relevant

5. Read the abstract (summary)

6. If available, access the full text

Search Tips:

- Use quotation marks for exact phrases: "fenbendazole" "cancer"
- Combine terms: fenbendazole AND cancer
- Exclude terms: fenbendazole cancer NOT veterinary
- Use filters to narrow by date, article type, etc.

Reading a Scientific Paper

Scientific papers follow a standard structure:

Abstract: Summary of the entire paper

- Start here to decide if the paper is relevant
- Tells you the question, methods, results, and conclusions

Introduction: Background and rationale

- Explains why the research was done
- Reviews previous research
- States the hypothesis or research question

Methods: How the research was conducted

- Critical for evaluating quality
- Should be detailed enough to replicate
- Look for appropriate controls and sample sizes

Results: What the researchers found

- Presents data, often with figures and tables
- Should be objective, without interpretation

Discussion: What the results mean

- Authors interpret their findings
- Compare to previous research
- Discuss limitations
- Suggest future research

References: Citations of other research

- Shows what previous work the study builds on
- Useful for finding related research

How to Read a Paper (Practical Approach)

You don't need to read every word. Here's an efficient approach:

1. **Read the abstract** - Does this paper address your question?
2. **Skim the introduction** - What's the background?
3. **Check the methods** - Was this well-designed research?
4. **Look at the figures and tables** - What are the key findings?
5. **Read the discussion** - What do the authors conclude?

6. **Note the limitations** - What are the caveats?

Evaluating Study Quality

Not all research is created equal. Here's what to look for:

Good Signs:

- Published in a reputable journal
- Appropriate sample size
- Proper controls (comparison groups)
- Randomization (for clinical trials)
- Blinding (researchers don't know who got what treatment)
- Statistical analysis
- Acknowledgment of limitations
- Funding from non-biased sources

Red Flags:

- Published in predatory or low-quality journals
- Very small sample size
- No control group
- Conflicts of interest not disclosed
- Overstated conclusions
- Cherry-picked data
- Methods not clearly described

Understanding Peer Review

Peer review is the process where other scientists evaluate research before publication:

How it works:

1. Researchers submit a paper to a journal
2. Editors send it to 2-3 expert reviewers
3. Reviewers evaluate methods, results, and conclusions
4. They recommend acceptance, revision, or rejection
5. Authors revise based on feedback
6. Paper is published if it meets standards

What peer review does:

- Catches obvious errors
- Ensures methods are sound
- Verifies that conclusions match data
- Maintains scientific standards

What peer review doesn't do:

- Guarantee the research is correct
- Detect fraud (usually)
- Ensure the research is important
- Make the paper easy to understand

Limitations of Peer Review:

- Reviewers may miss problems
- Bias can affect the process
- Negative results are less likely to be published
- It's not perfect, just the best system we have

Journal Quality Matters

Not all scientific journals are equal:

Top-Tier Journals (very selective, rigorous review):

- Nature, Science, Cell
- New England Journal of Medicine
- The Lancet, JAMA
- Cancer Cell, Cancer Research

Specialized Journals (respected in their fields):

- Journal of Clinical Oncology
- Cancer Letters
- Molecular Cancer Therapeutics
- Many others

Lower-Tier Journals (less selective):

- May have less rigorous review
- Still legitimate but less prestigious
- Findings should be viewed more cautiously

Predatory Journals (avoid):

- Publish almost anything for a fee
- Little or no peer review
- Designed to look legitimate
- Exploit researchers and mislead readers

How to Check Journal Quality:

- Look at the journal's impact factor (higher is generally better)
- Check if it's indexed in PubMed
- See if it's published by a reputable publisher
- Look for an editorial board of recognized experts

Interpreting Research Findings

Even when you find good research, interpreting it correctly is crucial:

Understanding Statistical Significance

You'll often see "$p < 0.05$" or "statistically significant" in papers. This means:

- The result is unlikely to be due to chance alone
- Specifically, less than 5% probability it's random
- But it doesn't tell you if the effect is large or clinically meaningful

Statistical significance ≠ clinical significance

A result can be statistically significant but clinically unimportant. For example:

- A drug extends survival by 2 days (statistically significant)
- But 2 days may not be meaningful to patients
- Context and magnitude matter

Understanding Effect Sizes

Look beyond p-values to effect sizes:

- How much did the treatment help?
- What percentage of patients responded?
- How large was the survival benefit?
- Are the effects clinically meaningful?

Relative Risk vs. Absolute Risk

This is a common source of confusion:

Relative risk: "50% reduction in risk"

- Sounds impressive
- But what was the baseline risk?

Absolute risk: "Risk decreased from 2% to 1%"

- Less impressive sounding
- But more informative

Example:

- "Fenbendazole reduced tumor growth by 50%" (relative)
- "Tumors grew 10mm instead of 20mm" (absolute)

Both statements might be true, but they give different impressions.

Confidence Intervals

These show the range of uncertainty:

- "Survival improved by 3 months (95% CI: 1-5 months)"
- This means we're 95% confident the true effect is between 1 and 5 months
- Wide confidence intervals indicate more uncertainty

Correlation vs. Causation (Again)

Even in research papers, correlation doesn't prove causation:

- Observational studies show associations
- But they can't prove one thing caused another
- Only randomized controlled trials can establish causation

Generalizability

Can results be applied to you?

Consider:

- Was the study in cells, animals, or humans?
- What type of cancer was studied?
- What stage of disease?
- What was the patient population?
- How similar are you to the study subjects?

Results in mice may not apply to humans. Results in one cancer type may not apply to another.

Red Flags in Health Claims

Certain phrases and patterns should immediately raise your skepticism:

Absolute Claims

- "Cures cancer"
- "100% effective"
- "Guaranteed results"
- "Works for everyone"

Reality: Nothing works for everyone. Legitimate treatments have response rates, not guarantees.

Conspiracy Theories

- "Doctors don't want you to know"
- "Big Pharma is suppressing this"
- "The medical establishment is hiding the cure"

Reality: While pharmaceutical companies do prioritize profits, thousands of independent researchers worldwide would love to find a cancer cure. Conspiracies of this scale are implausible.

Miracle Language

- "Miracle cure"
- "Breakthrough discovery"
- "Revolutionary treatment"
- "Secret remedy"

Reality: Real medical advances are incremental and carefully worded. Legitimate researchers don't use this language.

Anecdote-Heavy Claims

- "Thousands of people have been cured"
- "Everyone I know who tried this got better"
- "Amazing testimonials"

Reality: Anecdotes without data are unreliable. Where are the clinical trials?

Attacks on Conventional Medicine

- "Chemotherapy is poison"
- "Doctors just want your money"
- "Natural is always better"

Reality: Conventional medicine has limitations, but it's based on evidence. Attacking it doesn't make alternatives more effective.

Pressure Tactics

- "Act now before it's too late"
- "Limited time offer"
- "Don't wait for your doctor's approval"

Reality: Legitimate medical information doesn't pressure you. Take time to research and consult professionals.

Vague Mechanisms

- "Boosts your immune system"
- "Detoxifies your body"
- "Balances your energy"

Reality: Legitimate treatments have specific, testable mechanisms. Vague language often masks lack of evidence.

Cherry-Picked Evidence

- Citing only studies that support the claim
- Ignoring contradictory evidence
- Misrepresenting study findings

Reality: Honest evaluation presents all evidence, including limitations and negative findings.

The Role of Confirmation Bias

Confirmation bias is perhaps the biggest obstacle to evaluating information objectively. It's the tendency to:

- Seek out information that confirms what we already believe
- Interpret ambiguous evidence as supporting our beliefs
- Remember information that supports our views
- Discount information that contradicts our views

How Confirmation Bias Affects Cancer Patients

When you're facing cancer, confirmation bias is especially powerful:

If you believe fenbendazole works:

- You'll notice and remember success stories
- You'll interpret stable disease as "it's working"
- You'll attribute any improvement to fenbendazole

- You'll discount negative reports as "they didn't do it right"

If you're skeptical of fenbendazole:

- You'll focus on lack of clinical trials
- You'll emphasize risks and unknowns
- You'll attribute any improvement to conventional treatment
- You'll discount success stories as coincidence

Both perspectives involve bias. The goal is to recognize your bias and compensate for it.

Strategies to Counter Confirmation Bias

Actively seek contradictory information:

- Read skeptical perspectives
- Look for studies showing no effect
- Consider alternative explanations

Steel-man opposing arguments:

- Present the strongest version of views you disagree with
- Don't dismiss them with weak counterarguments
- Engage with the best evidence on both sides

Consider your emotional investment:

- Are you hoping fenbendazole works?
- Would you be disappointed if it doesn't?
- How might this affect your evaluation?

Use pre-commitment:

- Decide in advance what evidence would change your mind
- "I would stop believing fenbendazole works if..."
- This prevents moving the goalposts

Consult people who disagree:

- Talk to skeptics as well as believers
- Listen to their reasoning
- Don't dismiss them as closed-minded

Focus on process, not outcome:

- Evaluate the quality of evidence, not whether it supports your preferred conclusion
- Good evidence that contradicts your belief is more valuable than poor evidence that supports it

Social Media and Cancer Information

Social media has transformed how patients find and share health information. It offers benefits but also serious risks.

Benefits of Social Media

Community and Support:

- Connect with others facing similar challenges
- Share experiences and practical tips
- Emotional support and understanding

- Reduced isolation

Real-Time Information:

- Learn about new developments quickly
- Access patient experiences
- Find resources and recommendations

Patient Empowerment:

- Take active role in treatment decisions
- Learn from others' experiences
- Challenge medical paternalism

Risks of Social Media

Misinformation:

- Unverified claims spread rapidly
- No quality control
- Difficult to distinguish reliable from unreliable information

Echo Chambers:

- Algorithms show you content similar to what you've engaged with
- Creates bubbles where everyone agrees
- Dissenting views are filtered out

Emotional Manipulation:

- Dramatic stories get more engagement

- Fear and hope are powerful motivators
- Can lead to poor decisions

Scams and Exploitation:

- Vulnerable patients are targets
- Fake products and services
- Financial exploitation

Using Social Media Wisely

Join Moderated Groups:

- Look for groups with clear rules
- Moderators who remove misinformation
- Emphasis on evidence-based information

Verify Information:

- Don't believe everything you read
- Check claims against reliable sources
- Be especially skeptical of dramatic stories

Recognize Emotional Manipulation:

- Notice when content is designed to provoke fear or hope
- Step back and evaluate rationally
- Don't make decisions based on emotional posts

Protect Your Privacy:

- Be cautious about sharing personal health information

- Use privacy settings
- Be aware that posts are often permanent

Balance Online and Offline:

- Social media shouldn't replace medical care
- Discuss what you learn with your healthcare team
- Don't let online communities override professional advice

Be a Good Community Member:

- Share accurate information
- Be supportive without giving medical advice
- Acknowledge uncertainty
- Don't pressure others to follow your choices

Practical Exercise: Evaluating a Claim

Let's practice evaluating a hypothetical claim you might encounter:

Claim: "Fenbendazole cured my stage 4 lung cancer in 3 months! My tumors completely disappeared. Doctors are amazed. This is the cure they don't want you to know about!"

Step 1: Initial Reaction

- This is an extraordinary claim
- It uses red-flag language ("cure," "doctors don't want you to know")
- It's anecdotal (one person's experience)

Step 2: Questions to Ask

- What type of lung cancer? (Different types have different prognoses)
- What other treatments were used? (Chemotherapy? Immunotherapy?)
- What was the timeline? (When was diagnosis? When did treatment start?)
- How was response measured? (Scans? Biopsy? Symptoms?)
- What was the fenbendazole protocol? (Dose? Duration? Other supplements?)
- Who verified the results? (Oncologist? Independent radiologist?)

Step 3: Alternative Explanations

- Conventional treatment worked better than expected
- Misdiagnosis (wasn't actually stage 4)
- Spontaneous remission (rare but documented)
- Combination of factors
- Measurement error or misinterpretation of scans

Step 4: What Would Make This More Credible?

- Medical records and scan images
- Verification by independent oncologist
- Detailed timeline of all treatments

- Pathology reports confirming diagnosis
- Long-term follow-up (still cancer-free years later?)

Step 5: Appropriate Response

- Interesting case worth noting
- Cannot prove fenbendazole was responsible
- Doesn't establish that it would work for others
- Needs to be part of systematic data collection
- Should not be basis for treatment decisions alone

This kind of critical analysis should become automatic when you encounter health claims online.

Building Your Information Evaluation Skills

Like any skill, critical evaluation of health information improves with practice:

Start Small:

- Evaluate one claim or article per day
- Practice identifying red flags
- Check sources and citations

Keep a Journal:

- Record claims you encounter
- Note your initial reaction

- Document your evaluation process
- Track what you learn

Discuss with Others:

- Share what you're learning
- Get feedback on your reasoning
- Learn from others' perspectives

Consult Experts:

- Ask your healthcare team about claims you encounter
- Learn how they evaluate information
- Understand their reasoning

Stay Humble:

- Recognize the limits of your expertise
- Be willing to change your mind
- Acknowledge uncertainty

Continuous Learning:

- Your skills will improve over time
- Stay curious and skeptical
- Keep refining your approach

Key Takeaways

- The internet is full of health information, but quality varies enormously
- Critical thinking skills are essential for evaluating claims about fenbendazole or any treatment
- Extraordinary claims require extraordinary evidence—be especially skeptical of "miracle cure" language
- Anecdotes and testimonials, while compelling, cannot establish that a treatment works
- Scientific research papers are the gold standard, but they require skill to interpret correctly
- PubMed is a free, reliable resource for finding scientific research
- Peer review improves research quality but doesn't guarantee correctness
- Journal quality matters—not all publications are equally rigorous
- Statistical significance doesn't always mean clinical significance
- Red flags include absolute claims, conspiracy theories, pressure tactics, and attacks on conventional medicine
- Confirmation bias affects everyone—actively seek information that challenges your beliefs
- Social media offers community and support but also spreads

misinformation

- Develop a systematic approach to evaluating health claims
- When in doubt, consult qualified healthcare professionals
- Building evaluation skills takes practice but is one of the most valuable things you can do as a patient

CHAPTER EIGHT: CONVERSATIONS WITH YOUR HEALTHCARE TEAM

One of the most challenging aspects of considering fenbendazole is deciding whether and how to discuss it with your doctors. Many patients worry about their oncologist's reaction. Will they be dismissive? Angry? Supportive? Will it damage the doctor-patient relationship?

This chapter will help you navigate these conversations. We'll discuss why transparency matters, how to bring up fenbendazole, what questions to ask, and how to handle different responses from your healthcare team.

Why Transparency Matters

Let's start with the fundamental principle: you should tell your healthcare team about everything you're taking or considering taking. This includes fenbendazole, supplements, herbs, over-the-counter medications, and any other treatments.

Medical Safety

Your doctors need complete information to:

- **Avoid drug interactions**: Fenbendazole might interact with your cancer treatment or other medications
- **Interpret symptoms**: Side effects from fenbendazole could be mistaken for disease progression or treatment effects
- **Monitor appropriately**: Your doctor might order different tests if they know you're taking fenbendazole
- **Adjust treatment**: Some combinations might be dangerous or reduce effectiveness

Example: If you develop liver enzyme elevations, your doctor needs to know whether it could be from fenbendazole, chemotherapy, or both. Without this information, they might make incorrect treatment decisions.

Building Trust

Honesty strengthens the doctor-patient relationship:

- **Mutual respect**: Your doctor respects your autonomy; you respect their expertise
- **Open communication**: Transparency enables honest discussions
- **Collaborative decision-making**: You work together rather than at cross-purposes

- **Better care**: Your doctor can provide better guidance when they have complete information

Legal and Ethical Considerations

From a legal standpoint:

- **Informed consent**: Your doctor's recommendations are based on knowing your full treatment regimen
- **Liability**: If something goes wrong and your doctor didn't know about fenbendazole, it complicates matters
- **Medical records**: Complete records are important for continuity of care

The Risks of Secrecy

Some patients hide alternative treatments from their doctors. This can lead to:

- **Dangerous interactions**: Undetected drug interactions
- **Misdiagnosis**: Symptoms attributed to the wrong cause
- **Inappropriate treatment**: Decisions based on incomplete information
- **Damaged trust**: If your doctor discovers you've been hiding information
- **Worse outcomes**: Suboptimal care due to lack of information

Even if you think your doctor will disapprove, transparency is essential for your safety.

Preparing for the Conversation

Before talking to your oncologist about fenbendazole, prepare yourself:

Do Your Homework

- Read this book thoroughly
- Review the scientific research (especially the papers cited)
- Understand the limitations of the evidence
- Know what questions you want to ask
- Be prepared to explain why you're interested

Clarify Your Goals

What do you want from this conversation?

- **Information**: Learn your doctor's perspective
- **Permission**: Get approval to try fenbendazole
- **Monitoring**: Arrange appropriate safety monitoring
- **Integration**: Coordinate fenbendazole with conventional treatment
- **Support**: Maintain a good relationship with your doctor

Be clear about what you're asking for.

Manage Your Expectations

Realistically, your doctor might:

- Be unfamiliar with fenbendazole
- Be skeptical due to lack of clinical trials

- Be concerned about safety
- Be worried about false hope
- Be supportive but cautious
- Be completely opposed

Prepare for various responses.

Choose the Right Time

Don't bring this up:

- In a rushed appointment
- When discussing urgent medical issues
- When you're too emotional to have a rational discussion

Do bring it up:

- During a scheduled appointment with adequate time
- When your condition is stable
- When you're calm and prepared
- When you can have a thorough discussion

Bring Supporting Materials

Consider bringing:

- This book or key excerpts
- Copies of relevant research papers
- A written summary of what you've learned
- A list of questions

- Notes on your concerns and goals

Having materials shows you've done serious research, not just read Facebook posts.

How to Start the Conversation

The way you introduce the topic matters. Here are some approaches:

The Direct Approach

"Dr. Smith, I've been researching complementary approaches to my cancer treatment, and I'd like to discuss fenbendazole with you. I know it's not a standard treatment, but I've read about some interesting research. Can we talk about it?"

Pros: Clear, honest, respectful**Cons**: Might put doctor on defensive immediately

The Collaborative Approach

"Dr. Smith, I want to make sure I'm doing everything I can to fight this cancer. I've come across information about fenbendazole, and I'd value your expertise in helping me understand whether it might be worth considering. What do you know about it?"

Pros: Positions doctor as expert, invites collaboration**Cons**: Might seem manipulative if not genuine

The Informational Approach

"Dr. Smith, I've been reading about repurposed drugs for cancer, including fenbendazole. I'm not necessarily planning to take it, but I'm curious about your thoughts on the research. Have you heard about this?"

Pros: Low-pressure, genuinely seeking information**Cons**: Might not lead to actionable discussion

The Transparency Approach

"Dr. Smith, I need to be honest with you. I've been seriously considering trying fenbendazole based on some research I've read. Before I make any decisions, I want to discuss it with you and get your input."

Pros: Honest, shows respect for doctor's role**Cons**: Might seem like decision is already made

Choose the approach that feels most authentic to you and appropriate for your relationship with your doctor.

Questions to Ask Your Doctor

Come prepared with specific questions. Here are important ones:

About Fenbendazole Specifically

1. "Have you heard of patients using fenbendazole for cancer? What has been your experience?"

2. "Are you familiar with the research on fenbendazole and cancer? What's your assessment of the evidence?"

3. "Do you see any potential benefits to trying fenbendazole in my specific situation?"

4. "What are your concerns about fenbendazole, either in general or for my particular case?"

5. "Are there any specific risks I should be aware of given my type of cancer and current treatment?"

About Drug Interactions

1. "Could fenbendazole interact with my current chemotherapy/immunotherapy/targeted therapy?"

2. "Are there any medications I'm taking that might interact

with fenbendazole?"

3. "Could fenbendazole affect how my body processes my cancer treatment?"

4. "Should I avoid taking fenbendazole at certain times relative to my other treatments?"

About Monitoring and Safety

1. "If I were to try fenbendazole, what monitoring would you recommend?"

2. "What blood tests or scans should we do to check for side effects?"

3. "What symptoms should I watch for that might indicate a problem?"

4. "How often should I follow up with you if I'm taking fenbendazole?"

5. "At what point should I stop taking it if there are concerns?"

About Integration with Conventional Treatment

1. "Could fenbendazole interfere with the effectiveness of my standard treatment?"

2. "Might it enhance my standard treatment?"

3. "Should I wait until after my current treatment is complete, or could I start now?"

4. "Are there specific phases of treatment when fenbendazole would be more or less appropriate?"

About Alternatives and Options

1. "Are there other repurposed drugs or complementary approaches you'd recommend instead?"

2. "What would you suggest if I'm looking for additional ways to fight my cancer?"

3. "Are there any clinical trials I might be eligible for?"

About Your Doctor's Perspective

1. "What would you need to see to feel comfortable with me trying fenbendazole?"

2. "If you were in my situation, what would you do?"

3. "Can we agree on a plan for how to proceed, even if we don't fully agree on fenbendazole?"

About Documentation and Communication

1. "Will you document my use of fenbendazole in my medical records?"

2. "Should I inform my other doctors (surgeon, radiation oncologist, etc.) about this?"

3. "How should I communicate with you about my experience with fenbendazole?"

What Your Doctor Needs to Know

If you decide to use fenbendazole, your doctor needs specific information:

Before You Start

- **Your decision**: That you plan to try fenbendazole
- **Your reasoning**: Why you're interested (be honest)
- **Your source**: Where you'll obtain it
- **Your protocol**: Dose, frequency, formulation
- **Other supplements**: Everything else you're taking
- **Your expectations**: What you hope to achieve
- **Your commitment**: How long you plan to try it

During Use

- **Adherence**: Whether you're taking it as planned
- **Side effects**: Any symptoms or problems
- **Changes**: Any modifications to dose or schedule
- **Other treatments**: Any new supplements or treatments
- **Symptoms**: Any changes in your cancer symptoms
- **Concerns**: Any worries or questions

Ongoing

- **Results**: Your perception of whether it's helping
- **Scans and tests**: Your interpretation of results
- **Plans**: Whether you'll continue, stop, or modify
- **Other information**: Anything else relevant

Complete, ongoing communication is essential.

Possible Doctor Responses and How to Handle Them

Your doctor's response will vary. Here's how to handle different scenarios:

Response 1: "I'm Not Familiar with This"

This is common. Fenbendazole for cancer isn't mainstream, and most oncologists haven't studied it.

How to respond:

- Offer to share research papers
- Ask if they'd be willing to review the information
- Suggest they consult with colleagues
- Request a follow-up conversation after they've had time to research

What to say:"I understand this isn't something you've encountered before. I've brought some research papers that summarize the evidence. Would you be willing to review them and discuss this with me at my next appointment?"

Response 2: "There's No Evidence This Works"

This is technically true—there are no clinical trials in humans.

How to respond:

- Acknowledge the lack of clinical trials
- Mention the laboratory and animal research
- Explain that you understand the limitations
- Discuss your reasoning despite the uncertainty

What to say:"You're right that there are no clinical trials in humans. I understand that's a significant limitation. However, there is laboratory and animal research showing anti-cancer effects, and I'm aware of patient reports. Given my situation, I'm willing to accept the uncertainty. Can we discuss how to do this as safely as possible?"

Response 3: "This Could Be Dangerous"

Your doctor may have legitimate safety concerns.

How to respond:

- Ask for specific concerns
- Discuss the safety data from veterinary use
- Propose monitoring to detect problems early
- Show you're taking safety seriously

What to say:"I appreciate your concern for my safety. Can you tell me specifically what risks you're worried about? I'd like to understand your concerns and discuss how we might monitor for problems. What tests or monitoring would make you more comfortable?"

Response 4: "This Will Give You False Hope"

Doctors worry about patients pinning hopes on unproven treatments.

How to respond:

- Acknowledge the uncertainty
- Explain that you have realistic expectations
- Emphasize you're not abandoning conventional treatment
- Discuss how you'll evaluate whether it's working

What to say:"I understand your concern about false hope. I'm not expecting a miracle, and I'm not planning to stop my standard treatment. I see this as a potential additional tool, and I'll evaluate it realistically based on my scans and symptoms. I'm prepared for the possibility that it won't help."

Response 5: "I Can't Recommend This"

Many doctors won't recommend fenbendazole due to lack of evidence.

How to respond:

- Acknowledge their position
- Ask if they'll support your decision even if they don't recommend it
- Propose a compromise (monitoring without endorsement)
- Respect their professional boundaries

What to say:"I understand you can't recommend something without clinical trial evidence. I respect that. However, I'm considering trying this on my own. Would you be willing to monitor me and help keep me safe, even if you don't endorse the decision? I value your expertise and want to stay under your care."

Response 6: "Absolutely Not—I Forbid It"

Some doctors take a hard line against unproven treatments.

How to respond:

- Stay calm and respectful
- Ask for their specific concerns
- Explain your perspective
- Consider whether this doctor is right for you

What to say:"I hear that you're strongly opposed to this. Can you help me understand your concerns? I'm trying to make an informed decision, and your perspective is important to me. However, I also need to feel that I have some autonomy in my treatment decisions. Can we find a way to work together?"

If the relationship is damaged:

- Consider seeking a second opinion
- Look for a more collaborative doctor
- Don't let one doctor's opposition stop you from getting good care

Response 7: "Let's Try It and See"

Some doctors are open-minded and willing to support patient choices.

How to respond:

- Express appreciation
- Establish clear monitoring plan
- Set expectations for communication
- Document the plan

What to say:"Thank you for being open to this. I really appreciate your willingness to work with me. Let's establish a clear plan for monitoring and communication. What tests should we do, and how often should I follow up with you?"

Finding Supportive Doctors

If your current oncologist is completely opposed to fenbendazole and unwilling to monitor you, you might need to find a more supportive doctor.

Types of Doctors Who Might Be More Open

Integrative Oncologists:

- Combine conventional and complementary approaches
- More familiar with repurposed drugs and supplements
- Often more open to patient preferences
- May be more expensive (some don't take insurance)

Naturopathic Oncologists:

- Licensed naturopathic doctors specializing in cancer
- Focus on natural and complementary approaches
- Work alongside conventional oncologists
- Not available in all states

Functional Medicine Doctors:

- Focus on underlying causes and whole-person care
- Often more open to repurposed drugs
- May or may not specialize in cancer
- Variable training and credentials

Open-Minded Conventional Oncologists:

- Some conventional oncologists are open to patient experimentation

- They may not recommend fenbendazole but will monitor you
- Look for doctors who practice shared decision-making

How to Find Supportive Doctors

- Ask in online patient communities
- Search for "integrative oncology" in your area
- Contact cancer centers with integrative medicine programs
- Ask for referrals from other patients
- Interview potential doctors about their philosophy

Questions to Ask Potential Doctors

1. "What's your approach to patients who want to try complementary treatments?"
2. "Have you worked with patients using repurposed drugs like fenbendazole?"
3. "How do you balance evidence-based medicine with patient autonomy?"
4. "Would you be willing to monitor me if I choose to try fenbendazole?"
5. "How do you handle situations where you disagree with a patient's choice?"

Red Flags

Avoid doctors who:

- Promise cures or guaranteed results
- Discourage all conventional treatment
- Sell products or supplements in their office
- Make extreme claims
- Pressure you to follow their protocol
- Dismiss your concerns or questions

If Your Doctor Says No: Understanding Their Concerns

When doctors oppose fenbendazole, they usually have legitimate reasons:

Concern 1: Lack of Evidence

Doctors are trained to practice evidence-based medicine. Without clinical trials, they can't know:

- If fenbendazole works
- What dose is effective
- What side effects to expect
- How it interacts with other treatments

Their perspective: "I can't recommend something that hasn't been proven safe and effective in humans."

Your response: Acknowledge this concern while explaining your reasoning for accepting uncertainty.

Concern 2: Potential Harm

Even if fenbendazole seems safe, doctors worry about:

- Unknown side effects
- Drug interactions
- Interference with proven treatments
- Delayed diagnosis of problems

Their perspective: "First, do no harm. I can't risk your health on an unproven treatment."

Your response: Discuss monitoring and safety measures to minimize risks.

Concern 3: False Hope

Doctors see patients suffer when unproven treatments fail. They worry:

- You'll be disappointed
- You'll waste precious time
- You'll spend money on something ineffective
- You'll delay or refuse proven treatments

Their perspective: "I don't want you to pin your hopes on something unlikely to work."

Your response: Demonstrate realistic expectations and commitment to conventional treatment.

Concern 4: Professional Liability

Doctors face legal and professional risks:

- If something goes wrong, they could be sued
- Professional boards might question their judgment
- Colleagues might criticize them

- Insurance might not cover complications

Their perspective: "I could face serious consequences if I support this and something bad happens."

Your response: Acknowledge their position and consider signing a waiver or informed consent document.

Concern 5: Slippery Slope

Doctors worry that supporting one unproven treatment opens the door to others:

- Where do they draw the line?
- What about more dangerous alternatives?
- How do they maintain standards?

Their perspective: "If I support fenbendazole, what's next? Coffee enemas? Laetrile?"

Your response: Distinguish fenbendazole (which has scientific rationale) from treatments with no plausible mechanism.

Understanding vs. Agreement

You don't have to agree with your doctor's concerns, but understanding them helps you:

- Have more productive conversations
- Find compromises
- Maintain the relationship
- Make informed decisions

Second Opinions and Multidisciplinary Consultations

If you're struggling with your doctor's response, consider getting additional perspectives:

When to Seek a Second Opinion

- Your doctor is completely opposed and won't discuss it
- You feel your concerns aren't being heard
- You want expert input on your specific situation
- You're considering major treatment decisions
- You want to explore all options

How to Seek a Second Opinion

1. **Ask your current doctor**: Many will support this and provide records
2. **Contact major cancer centers**: They often have second opinion programs
3. **Look for specialists**: In your cancer type or integrative oncology
4. **Prepare thoroughly**: Bring all records, scans, and pathology reports
5. **Ask specific questions**: About fenbendazole and your overall treatment plan

Multidisciplinary Consultations

Consider assembling a team:

- **Medical oncologist**: Manages chemotherapy and overall care

- **Radiation oncologist**: If radiation is part of your treatment
- **Surgeon**: If surgery is an option
- **Integrative oncologist**: Advises on complementary approaches
- **Palliative care specialist**: Manages symptoms and quality of life
- **Nutritionist**: Optimizes diet during treatment

This team approach ensures comprehensive care and multiple perspectives.

Building a Collaborative Healthcare Team

The ideal scenario is a healthcare team that:

- Respects your autonomy
- Provides expert guidance
- Monitors you carefully
- Communicates openly
- Works together on your behalf

Principles of Collaboration

Mutual Respect:

- You respect their expertise
- They respect your autonomy

- Both parties listen to each other

Open Communication:

- You share complete information
- They explain their reasoning
- Both ask questions

Shared Decision-Making:

- You discuss options together
- You weigh pros and cons
- You make informed choices

Flexibility:

- Plans can be adjusted
- New information is incorporated
- Both parties remain open-minded

Common Goals:

- Focus on your health and wellbeing
- Work toward the best possible outcome
- Support each other in this effort

Your Role in the Team

As a patient, you contribute by:

- Being honest and transparent
- Doing your homework

- Asking good questions
- Following through on plans
- Communicating changes or concerns
- Respecting professional boundaries
- Being realistic about expectations

Your Doctor's Role

Your healthcare team contributes by:

- Providing expert medical guidance
- Monitoring your health
- Ordering appropriate tests
- Adjusting treatment as needed
- Being available for questions
- Respecting your autonomy
- Supporting your decisions when possible

Documenting Your Conversations

Keep records of your discussions about fenbendazole:

What to Document

- Date and time of conversation
- Who was present

- What you discussed
- Your doctor's concerns and recommendations
- Your questions and their answers
- Decisions made
- Follow-up plans

Why Documentation Matters

- Helps you remember details
- Provides a record if disputes arise
- Useful for other doctors
- Important for continuity of care
- May be relevant for insurance or legal issues

How to Document

- Take notes during appointments
- Ask if you can record conversations (with permission)
- Request written summaries from your doctor
- Keep a health journal
- Store documents securely

When the Relationship Isn't Working

Sometimes, despite best efforts, the doctor-patient relationship breaks down:

Signs of a Problematic Relationship

- Your doctor dismisses your concerns
- You feel judged or criticized
- Communication is poor
- You don't trust their judgment
- They won't listen to your preferences
- You're afraid to be honest with them

When to Consider Changing Doctors

- The relationship is causing you stress
- You're not getting good care
- Your doctor is unwilling to work with you
- You've tried to improve things without success
- You've lost confidence in them

How to Change Doctors

1. **Find a new doctor first**: Don't leave until you have somewhere to go
2. **Transfer records**: Request copies of all your medical records
3. **Be professional**: Don't burn bridges

4. **Explain briefly**: You can say you're seeking a different approach

5. **Don't feel guilty**: You have the right to choose your healthcare team

Maintaining Continuity

When changing doctors:

- Ensure new doctor has complete records
- Explain your treatment history
- Discuss your use of fenbendazole
- Establish clear communication
- Set expectations

Key Takeaways

- Transparency with your healthcare team is essential for your safety and the quality of your care
- Prepare thoroughly before discussing fenbendazole with your doctor
- Come with specific questions and be ready for various responses
- Your doctor needs to know what you're taking, how much, and why
- Doctors who oppose fenbendazole usually have legitimate

concerns based on lack of evidence and potential risks

- Understanding your doctor's perspective helps you have more productive conversations
- If your current doctor is completely opposed, consider seeking a second opinion or finding a more supportive doctor
- The ideal healthcare team respects your autonomy while providing expert guidance
- Document your conversations and decisions
- If the doctor-patient relationship isn't working, you have the right to find a new doctor
- Collaboration, mutual respect, and open communication are the foundations of good medical care
- Your healthcare team should support you in making informed decisions, even if they don't always agree with your choices

CHAPTER NINE: SOURCING, DOSING, AND FORMULATIONS

If you decide to try fenbendazole, you'll face practical questions: Where do I get it? What form should I use? How much should I take? How much will it cost? This chapter addresses these practical considerations.

Before we begin, an important disclaimer: This chapter provides information about what patients are doing, not medical advice about what you should do. Fenbendazole is not approved for human use in cancer treatment. Any use is off-label and experimental. Consult with qualified healthcare providers before making decisions.

Where Fenbendazole Comes From

Fenbendazole is manufactured as a veterinary antiparasitic drug. It's used to treat worms and parasites in:

- Dogs and cats
- Horses
- Cattle and livestock
- Other animals

Because it's a veterinary drug, you won't find it at your local pharmacy with a prescription. Instead, patients obtain it through various channels.

Veterinary Supply Stores

Physical stores that sell animal health products:

Pros:

- Can see product before buying
- Immediate availability
- Can ask questions in person

Cons:

- Limited selection
- May be more expensive
- Staff may question why you're buying it
- Not available in all areas

Online Veterinary Suppliers

Websites that sell animal health products:

Pros:

- Wide selection
- Competitive prices
- Convenient
- Discreet

Cons:

- Can't verify product before purchase
- Shipping time
- Quality varies by supplier
- Some sites are more reputable than others

Popular brands patients use include:

- Panacur (brand name)
- Safe-Guard (brand name)
- Generic fenbendazole products

Compounding Pharmacies

Some compounding pharmacies will make fenbendazole capsules for humans:

Pros:

- Pharmaceutical-grade quality
- Precise dosing
- Made for human consumption
- Professional oversight

Cons:

- Requires a prescription (some doctors will provide)
- More expensive
- Not all compounding pharmacies will do this
- Availability varies by location

International Sources

Some patients order from overseas:

Pros:

- May be cheaper
- Different formulations available
- Some countries sell it for human use

Cons:

- Quality concerns
- Customs issues
- Long shipping times
- Legal gray area
- No recourse if there's a problem

Quality and Purity Concerns

This is critical: veterinary products are not manufactured to pharmaceutical standards for human use.

Potential Issues:

Purity: Veterinary products may contain:

- Impurities from manufacturing
- Inactive ingredients not suitable for humans
- Contaminants
- Variable amounts of active ingredient

Consistency: Batch-to-batch variation may be greater than pharmaceutical products

Labeling: Dosing information is for animals, not humans

Storage: May not have been stored properly

Expiration: May be past expiration date

How to Minimize Quality Concerns:

1. **Buy from reputable suppliers**: Established companies with good reviews
2. **Check expiration dates**: Don't use expired products
3. **Look for lot numbers**: Indicates quality control
4. **Store properly**: Follow storage instructions
5. **Inspect products**: Look for signs of damage or tampering
6. **Consider compounding pharmacies**: If you can get a prescription

Third-Party Testing

Some patients have sent veterinary fenbendazole products for independent testing:

- Results generally show products contain what they claim
- Purity is usually acceptable

- Some variation between brands
- Testing is expensive and not always accessible

Different Formulations

Fenbendazole comes in several forms, each with advantages and disadvantages:

Granules/Powder (Most Common)

This is the most widely available form, sold for deworming dogs and horses.

Appearance: Fine white or off-white powder, sometimes in packets

Typical packaging:

- Individual packets (often 1 gram or 4 grams)
- Larger containers

Pros:

- Widely available
- Relatively inexpensive
- Easy to measure
- Can be mixed with food or drinks

Cons:

- Taste (bitter, unpleasant)
- Messy to handle
- Need to measure doses

- Contains inactive ingredients (flavoring for animals)

How patients use it:

- Mix with yogurt, applesauce, or smoothies
- Put in capsules (empty gelatin capsules available online)
- Mix with honey or nut butter
- Dissolve in water (doesn't dissolve well)

Practical tips:

- Use a small digital scale for accurate measuring
- Mix with strong-flavored foods to mask taste
- Take with fatty food (improves absorption)
- Store in a cool, dry place

Liquid Suspension

Some products come as a liquid suspension.

Appearance: White or off-white liquid

Pros:

- Easy to measure with syringe or dropper
- No mixing required
- May be easier to swallow

Cons:

- Less common
- Taste may be unpleasant

- Requires shaking before use
- Shorter shelf life once opened

How patients use it:

- Measure with oral syringe
- Mix with juice or other liquids
- Take directly (if tolerable)

Paste (for Horses)

Fenbendazole paste is sold for horses.

Appearance: Thick paste in a syringe-like applicator

Pros:

- Pre-measured doses
- Convenient
- Long shelf life

Cons:

- Designed for horses (very large doses)
- Difficult to measure small amounts accurately
- Unpleasant taste and texture
- Contains horse-specific flavoring

How patients use it:

- Squeeze out small amounts
- Mix with food

- Not recommended due to dosing difficulties

Compounded Capsules

Made by compounding pharmacies specifically for human use.

Appearance: Standard capsules, various sizes

Pros:

- Pharmaceutical quality
- Precise dosing
- Easy to take
- No taste
- Made for humans

Cons:

- Requires prescription
- More expensive
- Not widely available
- Insurance won't cover

Typical cost: $50-150 per month depending on dose and pharmacy

How to get them:

- Ask your doctor for a prescription
- Find a compounding pharmacy (not all will do this)
- Specify dose and quantity
- Pick up like any prescription

Dosing Information

This is perhaps the most uncertain aspect of using fenbendazole for cancer. There are no established human doses, no clinical trials to guide dosing, and no official recommendations.

What we have instead is:

- Doses used in animal studies
- Doses patients are using based on anecdotal reports
- Theoretical calculations based on animal data
- Individual experimentation

Important Disclaimer: The following information describes what patients are doing, not what you should do. Dosing should be discussed with a healthcare provider who knows your specific situation.

Common Patient Protocols

Based on online patient communities and reports, here are protocols patients commonly use:

The "Joe Tippens Protocol":

- 222 mg fenbendazole daily
- Taken for 3 consecutive days
- 4 days off
- Repeat weekly cycle

This is the most commonly cited protocol, based on Joe Tippens' experience.

Daily Dosing:

- 222-300 mg daily
- Taken continuously without breaks
- Some patients use 200 mg, others 300 mg

Higher Dose Protocols:

- 500-1000 mg daily
- Usually taken continuously
- Less common
- Based on animal study doses

Lower Dose Protocols:

- 100-150 mg daily
- For smaller individuals or cautious approach
- Less commonly reported

Pulse Dosing:

- Higher doses (500-1000 mg) for 3-5 days
- Followed by 2-4 weeks off
- Repeat cycle
- Less common

Factors Affecting Dose Choice

Patients consider various factors when choosing a dose:

Body Weight:

- Larger individuals may use higher doses
- Smaller individuals may use lower doses
- Some calculate based on mg/kg body weight

Cancer Type and Stage:

- More aggressive cancers might prompt higher doses
- Earlier stage might use lower doses
- No evidence to support these choices

Tolerance:

- Start low and increase if well-tolerated
- Reduce if side effects occur

Concurrent Treatments:

- May use lower doses with chemotherapy
- May use higher doses as monotherapy

Personal Philosophy:

- Some prefer "more is better"
- Others prefer "minimum effective dose"

Timing of Doses

With or Without Food:

Fenbendazole is fat-soluble, meaning it's better absorbed with fatty food.

Patients typically take it:

- With a meal containing fat

- With a spoonful of peanut butter or coconut oil
- With full-fat yogurt

Taking it on an empty stomach results in lower blood levels.

Time of Day:

No evidence suggests one time is better than another. Patients choose based on:

- Convenience
- When they remember
- When they eat fatty meals
- Personal preference

Consistency:

Taking it at the same time each day may help with:

- Remembering to take it
- Maintaining steady blood levels
- Tracking effects

Duration of Use

How long should someone take fenbendazole? There's no clear answer.

Patients typically:

- Continue as long as they perceive benefit
- Stop if scans show progression
- Take breaks periodically

- Continue indefinitely if stable

Considerations:

- Long-term safety is unknown
- Tolerance may develop
- Financial cost
- Quality of life impact

Dose Adjustments

Patients may adjust doses based on:

Response:

- Increase if no response after several months
- Decrease if stable and concerned about long-term use

Side Effects:

- Reduce dose if side effects occur
- Stop temporarily if serious side effects
- Resume at lower dose once resolved

Concurrent Treatments:

- May reduce during intensive chemotherapy
- May increase during treatment breaks

Lab Results:

- Reduce if liver enzymes elevate
- Adjust based on blood counts

Measuring Doses

For powder/granule formulations, accurate measurement is important:

Digital Scale:

- Most accurate method
- Measure in milligrams
- Calibrate regularly
- Use clean, dry surface

Pre-Measured Packets:

- Some products come in 1g or 4g packets
- Divide as needed
- Less precise but convenient

Volumetric Measurement:

- Less accurate
- Powder density varies
- Not recommended

Capsule Filling:

Many patients put powder into empty capsules:

Supplies needed:

- Empty gelatin or vegetarian capsules (size 00 or 0)
- Capsule filling machine (optional but helpful)
- Small funnel or scoop

- Digital scale

Process:

1. Weigh out desired dose
2. Separate capsule halves
3. Fill with powder
4. Close capsule
5. Store in cool, dry place

Tips:

- Size 00 capsules hold about 500-700 mg
- Size 0 capsules hold about 300-500 mg
- Tap capsule to settle powder
- Don't overfill (capsule won't close)

Cost Considerations

Fenbendazole is relatively inexpensive compared to cancer drugs, but costs vary:

Veterinary Products:

Granules/Powder:

- $20-50 for 1-3 months supply
- Depends on dose and brand
- Bulk purchases may be cheaper

Example: A box of three 4-gram packets (12 grams total) costs about $30-40. At 222 mg/day, this is about a 2-month supply.

Liquid Suspension:

- $30-60 for 1-2 months supply
- More expensive per dose than powder

Compounded Capsules:

- $50-150 per month
- Depends on dose and pharmacy
- Most expensive option
- Insurance won't cover

Long-Term Costs:

At 222 mg daily using veterinary powder:

- Monthly cost: $15-25
- Annual cost: $180-300

At 500 mg daily using compounded capsules:

- Monthly cost: $100-150
- Annual cost: $1,200-1,800

Additional Costs:

Don't forget:

- Supplements (if following a protocol with vitamins, etc.)
- Lab monitoring (blood tests)
- Doctor visits

- Shipping costs

Financial Assistance:

Unlike prescription drugs, there are no patient assistance programs for veterinary fenbendazole. However:

- Veterinary products are relatively affordable
- Generic versions are available
- Bulk buying may reduce costs
- Some online suppliers offer discounts

Insurance Coverage:

- Insurance will not cover veterinary fenbendazole
- Compounded prescriptions are usually not covered
- Lab monitoring may be covered if ordered by your doctor
- Some HSA/FSA accounts might reimburse (check your plan)

The Legal and Regulatory Situation

The legal status of using veterinary fenbendazole for human cancer treatment is complex and varies by jurisdiction.

In the United States:

Legal Status:

- Fenbendazole is not approved by the FDA for human use
- It's legal to purchase veterinary fenbendazole

- Using it for yourself is not illegal (off-label use)
- Doctors can prescribe it off-label (though most won't)

Regulatory Issues:

- FDA could theoretically take action against suppliers marketing it for human use
- Compounding pharmacies must follow state regulations
- Importing from overseas may face customs issues

Liability:

- Manufacturers are not liable for off-label human use
- Doctors who prescribe it assume some liability
- You assume risk by using it

In Other Countries:

Regulations vary:

- Some countries are more restrictive
- Some allow easier access
- Some have different formulations available
- Check your local laws

Customs and Importing:

If ordering internationally:

- May be seized by customs
- May be legal to import for personal use

- Regulations vary by country
- Large quantities may raise questions

The "Contraband" Issue

Some patients refer to fenbendazole as "contraband" because:

- It's not approved for human use
- There's a gray area in regulations
- Some feel they're doing something illicit

However:

- It's not actually contraband in most places
- Purchasing veterinary products is legal
- Off-label use is common in medicine
- The term is more emotional than legal

Protecting Yourself Legally:

- Keep records of your research and decision-making
- Document discussions with your doctor
- Don't make medical claims when purchasing
- Be honest with healthcare providers
- Understand you're assuming risk

Storage and Handling

Proper storage ensures fenbendazole remains effective:

Storage Conditions:

Temperature:

- Store at room temperature (68-77°F / 20-25°C)
- Avoid extreme heat or cold
- Don't refrigerate unless specified

Moisture:

- Keep in a dry place
- Moisture can degrade the powder
- Use airtight containers

Light:

- Store in original container or opaque container
- Protect from direct sunlight
- Light can degrade some drugs

Shelf Life:

Unopened:

- Check expiration date on package
- Usually 2-3 years from manufacture
- Store properly to maintain potency

Opened:

- Use within 6-12 months
- Reseal container tightly after each use

- Consider transferring to smaller containers to minimize air exposure
- Label with opening date

Signs of Degradation:

Watch for signs that fenbendazole may have degraded:

- Color change (yellowing or darkening)
- Clumping or caking of powder
- Unusual odor
- Moisture in container
- Past expiration date

If you notice any of these signs, discard the product and obtain fresh supply.

Handling Safety:

While fenbendazole is generally considered safe, practice good handling:

For Powder/Granules:

- Avoid inhaling powder
- Wash hands after handling
- Clean up spills promptly
- Keep away from children and pets
- Don't eat, drink, or smoke while handling

For All Formulations:

- Keep in original or labeled container
- Store out of reach of children
- Don't transfer to unmarked containers
- Dispose of properly (don't flush down toilet)

Travel Considerations:

If traveling with fenbendazole:

- Keep in original packaging if possible
- Bring documentation of your research
- Be prepared to explain if questioned
- Check regulations for your destination
- Pack in carry-on to control temperature
- Bring extra in case of delays

Disposal:

When disposing of expired or unused fenbendazole:

- Don't flush down toilet or drain
- Don't throw in regular trash if possible
- Check for medication take-back programs
- Mix with undesirable substance (coffee grounds, cat litter) in sealed bag
- Remove personal information from packaging

Key Takeaways

- Fenbendazole is available from veterinary suppliers, online sources, and compounding pharmacies
- Quality and purity vary—buy from reputable sources and check expiration dates
- Common formulations include powder/granules (most popular), liquid suspension, paste, and compounded capsules
- Dosing is uncertain—patients commonly use 200-300 mg daily, but there's no established human dose
- The "Joe Tippens Protocol" (222 mg for 3 days, 4 days off) is widely followed but not scientifically validated
- Always take with fatty food to improve absorption
- Costs range from $15-25/month for veterinary powder to $100-150/month for compounded capsules
- Using veterinary fenbendazole for human cancer treatment is legal in most places but not FDA-approved
- Proper storage (cool, dry, dark) maintains potency
- Accurate measurement using a digital scale is important for powder formulations
- All use is experimental and should be discussed with healthcare providers

- Document your protocol, sources, and any changes you make

CHAPTER TEN: MANAGING SIDE EFFECTS AND MONITORING

If you decide to use fenbendazole, understanding potential side effects and establishing appropriate monitoring is crucial for your safety. While fenbendazole appears to be well-tolerated based on veterinary use and patient reports, we lack systematic human safety data for cancer treatment doses.

This chapter covers what's known about side effects, how to monitor for problems, when to seek medical attention, and how to manage any issues that arise.

What We Know About Side Effects

Our knowledge of fenbendazole side effects in humans comes from several sources:

Veterinary Data:

- Decades of use in animals at antiparasitic doses
- Generally well-tolerated with minimal side effects
- Occasional gastrointestinal upset
- Rare liver enzyme elevations

Accidental Human Exposure:

- Veterinarians and farmers occasionally exposed
- Few reported problems
- Limited systematic data

Patient Reports:

- Self-reported experiences from cancer patients
- Variable doses and durations
- Often concurrent with other treatments
- Selection bias (people with problems may be more or less likely to report)

Related Drugs:

- Mebendazole (similar drug) used in humans
- Generally well-tolerated
- Provides some guidance on what to expect

Common Side Effects Reported by Patients

Based on patient reports in online communities, here are side effects that some people experience:

Gastrointestinal Effects (Most Common):

Nausea:

- Mild to moderate in some patients
- Often improves after first few doses
- May be worse on empty stomach
- Usually manageable

Diarrhea or Loose Stools:

- Reported by some patients
- Usually mild
- May be related to dose
- Often temporary

Stomach Discomfort:

- Mild cramping or bloating
- Usually resolves quickly
- Taking with food may help

Constipation:

- Less common than diarrhea
- May be related to other factors
- Usually mild

Taste Issues:

- Bitter taste if powder not encapsulated
- Aftertaste reported by some
- Easily managed by using capsules or mixing with strong-flavored foods

Fatigue and Energy Changes:

Increased Fatigue:

- Some patients report feeling more tired
- May be temporary
- Could be related to cancer or other treatments
- Difficult to attribute definitively to fenbendazole

"Die-Off" Reactions:

- Some patients report feeling worse initially
- Attributed to tumor cell death releasing contents
- Not scientifically verified
- Could be coincidental

Neurological Effects (Rare):

Headaches:

- Reported occasionally
- Usually mild
- May be unrelated to fenbendazole

Dizziness:

- Rarely reported
- Usually mild and transient

Neuropathy:

- Very rarely reported
- Tingling or numbness in hands/feet
- Could be related to chemotherapy rather than fenbendazole
- Should be evaluated by doctor

Liver-Related Effects:

Elevated Liver Enzymes:

- Detected on blood tests
- Usually mild
- May require dose reduction or discontinuation
- Typically reversible

Jaundice:

- Extremely rare
- Yellowing of skin or eyes
- Requires immediate medical attention

Allergic Reactions (Rare):

Rash or Itching:

- Occasionally reported

- Usually mild
- May indicate allergy

More Serious Reactions:

- Difficulty breathing
- Swelling of face, lips, or tongue
- Severe rash
- Require immediate medical attention

Blood-Related Effects:

Changes in Blood Counts:

- Rarely reported
- Could affect white blood cells, red blood cells, or platelets
- Requires monitoring
- May be related to cancer or other treatments

Less Common or Uncertain Side Effects

Some effects are reported but difficult to verify:

Mood Changes:

- Anxiety or depression
- Could be related to cancer diagnosis
- Difficult to attribute to fenbendazole

Sleep Disturbances:

- Insomnia or vivid dreams
- Reported by some patients
- May be coincidental

Skin Changes:

- Dry skin or minor rashes
- Usually mild
- Could have multiple causes

Hair or Nail Changes:

- Rarely reported
- Could be related to cancer or other treatments

Factors Affecting Side Effects

Several factors may influence whether you experience side effects:

Dose:

- Higher doses may cause more side effects
- Starting low and increasing gradually may improve tolerance

Individual Variation:

- People respond differently to medications
- Genetic factors affect drug metabolism
- Some people are more sensitive than others

Concurrent Treatments:

- Chemotherapy causes many side effects
- Difficult to determine what's causing what
- Interactions may increase side effects

Underlying Health:

- Liver or kidney problems may increase risk
- Other medical conditions matter
- Overall health status affects tolerance

Formulation:

- Veterinary products contain inactive ingredients
- These may cause reactions in some people
- Compounded formulations may be better tolerated

Monitoring: What Tests and When

Appropriate monitoring helps detect problems early. Work with your healthcare team to establish a monitoring plan.

Baseline Testing (Before Starting):

Establish baseline values before starting fenbendazole:

Blood Tests:

- Complete Blood Count (CBC): Checks red blood cells, white blood cells, platelets
- Comprehensive Metabolic Panel (CMP): Checks liver enzymes, kidney function, electrolytes

- Liver Function Tests (LFTs): AST, ALT, alkaline phosphatase, bilirubin

Other Baseline Assessments:

- Blood pressure
- Weight
- Symptom inventory
- Quality of life assessment
- Current medications and supplements list

Ongoing Monitoring:

How often to monitor depends on your situation, but general guidelines:

First Month:

- Blood tests every 2-4 weeks
- More frequent if you have pre-existing liver or kidney issues
- Watch for any new symptoms

After First Month:

- Blood tests every 4-8 weeks if stable
- More frequent if abnormalities detected
- Coordinate with your cancer monitoring schedule

What to Monitor:

Liver Function:

- AST and ALT (liver enzymes)

- Alkaline phosphatase
- Bilirubin
- Most important to watch

Blood Counts:

- White blood cells (immune function)
- Red blood cells (anemia)
- Platelets (clotting)

Kidney Function:

- Creatinine
- BUN (blood urea nitrogen)
- Less commonly affected but important

Other:

- Electrolytes
- Blood sugar (if diabetic)
- Any specific concerns based on your health

Cancer Monitoring:

Continue your regular cancer monitoring:

Scans:

- CT, MRI, or PET scans as scheduled
- Don't change your monitoring schedule
- Discuss results with your oncologist

Tumor Markers:

- If applicable to your cancer type
- CEA, CA 19-9, PSA, etc.
- Track trends over time

Physical Exams:

- Regular oncology appointments
- Report any new symptoms
- Don't skip appointments

Symptom Tracking:

Keep a detailed log:

Daily Tracking:

- Dose taken (amount, time)
- Any side effects
- Energy level
- Appetite
- Sleep quality
- Pain levels
- Other symptoms

Weekly Summary:

- Overall trends
- Any patterns

- Changes from previous week

Monthly Review:

- Compare to baseline
- Discuss with healthcare team
- Adjust protocol if needed

When to Seek Medical Attention

Know when to contact your doctor or seek emergency care:

Contact Your Doctor Soon (Within 24-48 Hours):

- Persistent nausea or vomiting
- Diarrhea lasting more than 2 days
- New or worsening fatigue
- Unexplained fever
- New pain
- Any concerning symptoms

Seek Immediate Medical Attention:

- Severe abdominal pain
- Yellowing of skin or eyes (jaundice)
- Dark urine or pale stools
- Difficulty breathing

- Chest pain
- Severe allergic reaction (rash, swelling, difficulty breathing)
- Severe headache or neurological symptoms
- Bleeding or bruising
- Signs of infection with fever

Emergency Room Situations:

- Difficulty breathing
- Chest pain
- Severe allergic reaction
- Loss of consciousness
- Severe bleeding
- Any life-threatening symptom

Don't hesitate to seek care if you're concerned. It's better to be cautious.

Managing Common Side Effects

Here are strategies for managing side effects if they occur:

For Nausea:

- Take with food
- Eat smaller, more frequent meals
- Avoid strong odors

- Try ginger tea or ginger supplements
- Stay hydrated
- Consider anti-nausea medication (discuss with doctor)
- Take at bedtime if nausea is problematic

For Diarrhea:

- Stay well hydrated
- Eat bland foods (BRAT diet: bananas, rice, applesauce, toast)
- Avoid dairy, caffeine, and fatty foods temporarily
- Consider probiotics
- Over-the-counter anti-diarrheal medication if needed (discuss with doctor)
- Reduce dose if persistent

For Fatigue:

- Get adequate rest
- Pace activities
- Light exercise if tolerated
- Good nutrition
- Stay hydrated
- Consider reducing dose
- Rule out other causes (anemia, thyroid, etc.)

For Stomach Discomfort:

- Take with food
- Avoid spicy or acidic foods
- Smaller, more frequent meals
- Antacids if needed (discuss timing with doctor)
- Reduce dose if persistent

For Headaches:

- Stay hydrated
- Over-the-counter pain relievers (acetaminophen, ibuprofen)
- Rest in quiet, dark room
- Reduce dose if persistent
- Rule out other causes

For Taste Issues:

- Use capsules instead of powder
- Mix powder with strong-flavored foods
- Brush teeth after taking
- Use mints or gum
- Drink flavored beverages

Dose Adjustments for Side Effects

If you experience side effects, consider these strategies:

Reduce Dose:

- Cut dose by 25-50%
- See if symptoms improve
- Gradually increase again if tolerated

Change Schedule:

- Take at different time of day
- Split dose into smaller amounts
- Try the 3-days-on, 4-days-off protocol if taking daily

Take a Break:

- Stop for a few days
- Let side effects resolve
- Restart at lower dose

Change Formulation:

- Switch from powder to capsules
- Try different brand
- Consider compounded version

Add Supportive Measures:

- Take with specific foods
- Add supplements to reduce side effects
- Adjust other medications (with doctor approval)

Drug Interactions and Contraindications

Be aware of potential interactions:

Possible Interactions:

Chemotherapy Drugs:

- May interact with some chemotherapy agents
- Discuss timing with oncologist
- May need to separate doses

Immunotherapy:

- Unknown interactions
- Theoretical concerns about immune effects
- Discuss with oncologist

Other Medications:

- Drugs metabolized by liver (many medications)
- Blood thinners (theoretical concern)
- Seizure medications
- Discuss all medications with doctor

Supplements:

- High-dose antioxidants may interfere with some cancer treatments
- Discuss all supplements with healthcare team

- Timing may matter

Contraindications (When NOT to Use):

Absolute Contraindications:

- Known allergy to benzimidazoles
- Severe liver disease
- Pregnancy (unless benefits clearly outweigh risks)

Relative Contraindications (Use with Caution):

- Moderate liver disease
- Kidney disease
- Bone marrow suppression
- Taking multiple medications
- Very young or very old age

Special Situations:

During Active Chemotherapy:

- Discuss timing with oncologist
- May need to avoid during certain chemotherapy cycles
- Monitor more closely

Before Surgery:

- Discuss with surgeon
- May need to stop temporarily
- Consider effects on healing

During Radiation:

- Unknown interactions
- Discuss with radiation oncologist
- May be beneficial or problematic

Laboratory Abnormalities: What They Mean

Understanding lab results helps you monitor safety:

Liver Enzymes (AST, ALT):

Normal: Usually less than 40 U/L (varies by lab)

Mild Elevation (1-2x normal):

- Monitor closely
- May continue with caution
- Recheck in 1-2 weeks

Moderate Elevation (2-3x normal):

- Consider dose reduction
- Recheck in 1 week
- May need to stop temporarily

Severe Elevation (>3x normal):

- Stop fenbendazole
- Seek medical evaluation
- Investigate other causes

White Blood Cell Count:

Normal: 4,000-11,000 cells/μL

Low (<4,000):

- May be from cancer or chemotherapy
- Monitor closely
- Consider dose reduction if declining
- Watch for infection

Platelet Count:

Normal: 150,000-400,000/μL

Low (<150,000):

- May be from cancer or chemotherapy
- Monitor closely
- Consider stopping if very low (<50,000)
- Watch for bleeding

Kidney Function (Creatinine):

Normal: 0.6-1.2 mg/dL

Elevated:

- May indicate kidney stress
- Ensure adequate hydration
- Consider dose reduction
- Investigate other causes

Long-Term Monitoring Considerations

For those using fenbendazole long-term:

Cumulative Effects:

- Unknown if long-term use causes cumulative toxicity
- Continue regular monitoring
- Watch for gradual changes

Tolerance:

- Body may adapt over time
- Effectiveness may change
- Side effects may improve or worsen

Periodic Breaks:

- Some patients take periodic breaks
- May reduce risk of cumulative effects
- No evidence on optimal schedule

Ongoing Assessment:

- Regularly reassess risk-benefit ratio
- Is it still worth taking?
- Are there signs of benefit?
- Are side effects manageable?

Working with Your Healthcare Team

Effective monitoring requires collaboration:

Communication:

- Report all side effects, even minor ones
- Bring your symptom log to appointments
- Ask questions about lab results
- Discuss any concerns

Coordination:

- Ensure all doctors know you're taking fenbendazole
- Coordinate monitoring with cancer care
- Avoid duplicate testing when possible
- Share results among your healthcare team

Documentation:

- Keep copies of all lab results
- Track trends over time
- Note any interventions and responses
- Maintain organized records

Adjustments:

- Be willing to adjust protocol based on monitoring
- Don't ignore warning signs
- Prioritize safety over continuing at all costs

Quality of Life Considerations

Monitor not just lab values but how you feel:

Physical Function:

- Energy levels
- Ability to do daily activities
- Exercise tolerance
- Sleep quality

Emotional Well-Being:

- Mood
- Anxiety levels
- Stress
- Overall outlook

Social Function:

- Relationships
- Work or activities
- Social engagement

Symptom Burden:

- Pain levels
- Other cancer symptoms
- Treatment side effects

- Overall comfort

If fenbendazole significantly reduces your quality of life, it may not be worth continuing, even if lab values are stable.

Key Takeaways

- Fenbendazole appears generally well-tolerated based on veterinary use and patient reports, but systematic human safety data is lacking
- Common side effects include mild gastrointestinal symptoms (nausea, diarrhea, stomach discomfort)
- Serious side effects are rare but can include liver enzyme elevations and allergic reactions
- Baseline blood tests (CBC, CMP, LFTs) should be done before starting
- Ongoing monitoring every 2-4 weeks initially, then every 4-8 weeks if stable
- Liver function tests are the most important to monitor
- Keep a detailed symptom log to track patterns and changes
- Know when to seek medical attention—don't ignore warning signs
- Most side effects can be managed with dose adjustments, timing changes, or supportive measures
- Discuss all medications and supplements with your health-

care team to avoid interactions

- Long-term safety is unknown—continue regular monitoring indefinitely
- Quality of life matters—if side effects significantly impact your well-being, reconsider whether to continue
- Work collaboratively with your healthcare team for safe monitoring
- Document everything and maintain organized records

CHAPTER ELEVEN: COMBINATION APPROACHES AND PROTOCOLS

Many patients using fenbendazole don't take it alone. They combine it with other supplements, repurposed drugs, dietary changes, and conventional treatments. This chapter explores common combination approaches, the rationale behind them, potential benefits and risks, and how to think about combinations safely.

Important Note: This chapter describes what patients are doing, not medical recommendations. All combinations should be discussed with qualified healthcare providers. Interactions and risks increase with each additional substance.

The Rationale for Combination Approaches

Why do patients combine fenbendazole with other interventions?

Multiple Mechanisms:

- Cancer is complex with multiple survival pathways
- Attacking through multiple mechanisms may be more effective
- Single agents rarely cure cancer alone

Synergy:

- Some combinations may work better together than separately
- Synergistic effects mean 1+1=3, not just 2
- Laboratory studies show synergy with some combinations

Overcoming Resistance:

- Cancer cells develop resistance to single agents
- Multiple agents may prevent or overcome resistance
- Different mechanisms reduce escape routes

Comprehensive Approach:

- Address cancer from multiple angles
- Support overall health while fighting cancer
- Optimize conditions for treatment success

Patient Empowerment:

- Taking multiple actions provides sense of control
- Addresses the desire to "do everything possible"

- May improve psychological well-being

The Joe Tippens Protocol

The most famous fenbendazole protocol includes several components:

Core Components:

1. **Fenbendazole**: 222 mg daily for 3 consecutive days, then 4 days off (weekly cycle)
2. **Vitamin E**: 800 IU daily (as tocopherols and tocotrienols)
    - Antioxidant properties
    - May enhance fenbendazole effects
    - Supports overall health
3. **Curcumin**: 600 mg daily (with bioperine for absorption)
    - Anti-inflammatory properties
    - May have anti-cancer effects
    - Enhances bioavailability of other compounds
4. **CBD Oil**: 25 mg daily
    - May have anti-cancer properties
    - Reduces anxiety and improves sleep
    - Anti-inflammatory effects

Rationale:

This protocol is based on Joe Tippens' personal experience, not scientific research. He took these supplements together and experienced cancer remission. However:

- We don't know which component(s) were responsible
- His conventional treatment may have been the key factor
- The combination may have worked synergistically
- It might have been coincidental

Variations:

Patients modify this protocol in various ways:

- Taking fenbendazole daily instead of 3-on-4-off
- Using different doses
- Adding or removing components
- Substituting similar supplements

Common Supplement Additions

Beyond the Tippens protocol, patients often add:

Berberine:

- Activates AMPK (energy sensor)
- May affect cancer metabolism
- Anti-inflammatory properties
- Typical dose: 500 mg 2-3 times daily

Alpha-Lipoic Acid:

- Antioxidant
- May enhance metabolic effects
- Supports mitochondrial function
- Typical dose: 600 mg daily

Milk Thistle (Silymarin):

- Liver support
- May protect against liver toxicity
- Antioxidant properties
- Typical dose: 150-300 mg daily

Omega-3 Fatty Acids:

- Anti-inflammatory
- May reduce cancer cachexia
- Supports overall health
- Typical dose: 2-4 grams EPA/DHA daily

Vitamin D:

- Immune support
- May have anti-cancer properties
- Many cancer patients are deficient
- Typical dose: 2,000-5,000 IU daily (check blood levels)

Probiotics:

- Gut health
- Immune support
- May reduce treatment side effects
- Various strains and doses

Melatonin:

- Antioxidant
- May have anti-cancer properties
- Improves sleep
- Typical dose: 3-20 mg at bedtime

Turkey Tail Mushroom (PSK/PSP):

- Immune support
- Some evidence in cancer treatment
- Generally safe
- Typical dose: varies by product

Other Repurposed Drugs

Some patients combine fenbendazole with other repurposed medications:

Metformin:

- Diabetes drug

- May affect cancer metabolism
- Some evidence of anti-cancer effects
- Requires prescription
- Typical dose: 500-1,000 mg twice daily

Mebendazole:

- Similar to fenbendazole
- Some patients use both or alternate
- May have slightly different properties
- Requires prescription in most countries

Doxycycline:

- Antibiotic
- May affect cancer stem cells
- Anti-inflammatory properties
- Requires prescription
- Typical dose: 100-200 mg daily

Statins:

- Cholesterol-lowering drugs
- May have anti-cancer properties
- Generally safe
- Requires prescription

Aspirin:

- Anti-inflammatory
- Some evidence of cancer prevention
- Blood-thinning effects
- Typical dose: 81-325 mg daily

Cimetidine (Tagamet):

- Heartburn medication
- May enhance immune response
- Some evidence in cancer treatment
- Available over-the-counter
- Typical dose: 800 mg daily

Important Considerations for Repurposed Drugs:

- All require medical supervision
- Potential for drug interactions
- Side effects and contraindications
- Need for monitoring
- Should not replace proven treatments

Dietary Approaches

Many patients combine fenbendazole with specific diets:

Ketogenic Diet:

Rationale:

- Cancer cells prefer glucose for energy
- Ketogenic diet restricts carbohydrates
- May "starve" cancer cells
- Forces body to use ketones for fuel

Components:

- Very low carbohydrate (20-50g daily)
- High fat (70-80% of calories)
- Moderate protein (15-20% of calories)

Considerations:

- Difficult to maintain
- May cause side effects (keto flu)
- Not suitable for everyone
- Limited evidence in humans
- Should be medically supervised

Fasting and Calorie Restriction:

Intermittent Fasting:

- Time-restricted eating (e.g., 16:8)
- May enhance autophagy
- Some evidence of benefits

- Generally safe for most people

Fasting Around Chemotherapy:

- Short fasts (24-48 hours) before/after chemo
- May protect normal cells
- Some evidence of benefits
- Must be medically supervised

Calorie Restriction:

- Reducing overall calorie intake
- May slow cancer growth
- Difficult to maintain
- Risk of malnutrition in cancer patients

Anti-Inflammatory Diet:

Components:

- Emphasis on vegetables and fruits
- Healthy fats (olive oil, omega-3s)
- Whole grains
- Lean proteins
- Minimal processed foods and sugar

Benefits:

- Reduces inflammation
- Supports overall health

- Generally safe and healthy
- May improve treatment tolerance

Alkaline Diet:

Rationale:

- Cancer cells create acidic environment
- Alkaline diet may counteract this
- Emphasis on vegetables, fruits, nuts

Considerations:

- Limited scientific evidence
- Body tightly regulates pH
- May be healthy but mechanism unclear

Supplements for Dietary Support:

- Digestive enzymes
- Protein powders (if appetite poor)
- Greens powders
- Multivitamins

Integration with Conventional Treatment

The most important combinations involve conventional cancer treatment:

With Chemotherapy:

Potential Benefits:

- May enhance chemotherapy effects
- Could reduce side effects
- Might prevent resistance

Potential Risks:

- Could interfere with chemotherapy
- May increase toxicity
- Unknown interactions

Considerations:

- Timing is crucial
- Discuss with oncologist
- May need to separate doses
- Close monitoring essential

Specific Chemotherapy Considerations:

Different chemotherapy drugs may interact differently:

- **Taxanes** (paclitaxel, docetaxel): Both affect microtubules—potential for synergy or increased toxicity
- **Platinum drugs** (cisplatin, carboplatin): Unknown interactions
- **Antimetabolites** (5-FU, gemcitabine): May have complementary mechanisms
- **Anthracyclines** (doxorubicin): Unknown interactions

With Immunotherapy:

Potential Benefits:

- May enhance immune response
- Could improve outcomes

Potential Risks:

- Unknown effects on immune system
- Could theoretically interfere

Considerations:

- Very limited data
- Discuss with oncologist
- Monitor for immune-related side effects

With Radiation Therapy:

Potential Benefits:

- May sensitize cancer cells to radiation
- Could enhance effectiveness

Potential Risks:

- Could increase radiation toxicity
- Unknown interactions

Considerations:

- Some laboratory evidence of benefit
- Timing may matter
- Discuss with radiation oncologist

With Targeted Therapy:

Potential Benefits:

- Different mechanisms may be complementary
- Could overcome resistance

Potential Risks:

- Unknown interactions
- May affect drug metabolism

Considerations:

- Depends on specific targeted therapy
- Discuss with oncologist
- Monitor closely

With Hormonal Therapy:

Potential Benefits:

- May work through different mechanisms
- Could be complementary

Potential Risks:

- Unknown interactions

Considerations:

- Generally lower risk than with chemotherapy
- Still requires discussion with oncologist

Timing Strategies

When combining multiple interventions, timing matters:

Separation Strategies:

Time of Day:

- Take fenbendazole at different time than other medications
- Morning vs. evening dosing
- With meals vs. between meals

Day of Week:

- Fenbendazole on certain days
- Other supplements on different days
- Chemotherapy on specific schedule

Cycling:

- Rotate different interventions
- Periods on and off various supplements
- May reduce tolerance and resistance

Pulsed Dosing:

- High-dose periods followed by breaks
- May maximize benefits while minimizing toxicity
- Used for some supplements and drugs

Chemotherapy Coordination:

Before Chemotherapy:

- Some patients stop fenbendazole 1-2 days before
- Concern about interference

- No evidence either way

During Chemotherapy:

- Some continue, some stop
- Individual decision with oncologist
- Consider type of chemotherapy

After Chemotherapy:

- Resume when blood counts recover
- May help with recovery
- Monitor closely

Potential Synergies

Some combinations may work better together:

Fenbendazole + Vitamin E:

- Vitamin E may enhance fenbendazole effects
- Antioxidant protection
- Part of Tippens protocol

Fenbendazole + Curcumin:

- Both affect multiple cancer pathways
- Anti-inflammatory effects
- May enhance absorption

Fenbendazole + Metformin:

- Both affect metabolism
- May have synergistic effects
- Some laboratory evidence

Fenbendazole + Berberine:

- Both activate AMPK
- Metabolic effects
- Theoretical synergy

Fenbendazole + CBD:

- May enhance anti-cancer effects
- Reduces anxiety
- Part of Tippens protocol

Fenbendazole + Ketogenic Diet:

- Both affect metabolism
- May "starve" cancer cells
- Theoretical synergy

Fenbendazole + Chemotherapy:

- May sensitize cancer cells
- Could overcome resistance
- Requires careful coordination

Potential Antagonisms

Some combinations might work against each other:

Antioxidants + Chemotherapy/Radiation:

Concern:

- High-dose antioxidants may protect cancer cells
- Could reduce treatment effectiveness
- Controversial topic

Evidence:

- Mixed research findings
- May depend on type and dose
- Timing may matter

Recommendations:

- Discuss with oncologist
- Consider stopping high-dose antioxidants during treatment
- Food-based antioxidants generally considered safe

Immune Stimulants + Immunotherapy:

Concern:

- Could overstimulate immune system
- May increase autoimmune side effects

Recommendations:

- Discuss with oncologist
- Monitor closely

- May need to avoid certain supplements

Multiple Liver-Metabolized Drugs:

Concern:

- Competition for liver enzymes
- May affect drug levels
- Increased toxicity risk

Recommendations:

- Discuss all medications with doctor
- Monitor liver function
- Consider timing strategies

Safety Considerations for Combinations

Adding multiple interventions increases complexity and risk:

Increased Monitoring Needs:

- More frequent blood tests
- Watch for unexpected interactions
- Track multiple variables

Cumulative Toxicity:

- Multiple substances may stress liver
- Kidney function may be affected
- Overall burden on body

Difficulty Attributing Effects:

- Hard to know what's helping
- Hard to know what's causing problems
- Makes adjustments challenging

Cost Considerations:

- Multiple supplements add up
- Monitoring costs increase
- May not be sustainable long-term

Complexity and Adherence:

- Difficult to remember multiple supplements
- Timing becomes complicated
- May reduce adherence to all interventions

Unknown Interactions:

- Most combinations haven't been studied
- Unexpected interactions possible
- Risk increases with each addition

A Rational Approach to Combinations

If considering combinations, approach systematically:

Start Simple:

- Begin with fenbendazole alone

- Assess tolerance and effects
- Add one thing at a time

Add Gradually:

- Introduce new interventions one at a time
- Wait 1-2 weeks between additions
- Monitor for changes

Prioritize:

- Focus on interventions with best evidence
- Consider risk-benefit ratio
- Don't add things just because others do

Document Everything:

- Keep detailed records
- Track what you're taking and when
- Note any changes or effects

Regular Reassessment:

- Periodically review your protocol
- Eliminate things that aren't helping
- Simplify when possible

Work with Healthcare Team:

- Discuss all additions
- Get input on safety

- Coordinate monitoring

Common Combination Protocols

Here are some protocols patients use (not recommendations):

Minimal Protocol:

- Fenbendazole alone
- Basic multivitamin
- Healthy diet
- Conventional treatment as prescribed

Tippens Protocol:

- Fenbendazole 222 mg (3 days on, 4 off)
- Vitamin E 800 IU daily
- Curcumin 600 mg daily
- CBD oil 25 mg daily

Metabolic Protocol:

- Fenbendazole 222-300 mg daily
- Metformin 500-1000 mg twice daily
- Berberine 500 mg three times daily
- Ketogenic or low-carb diet
- Intermittent fasting

Comprehensive Protocol:

- Fenbendazole 222-300 mg daily
- Multiple supplements (vitamin E, curcumin, CBD, berberine, etc.)
- Repurposed drugs (metformin, others)
- Dietary modifications
- Conventional treatment
- Lifestyle interventions

Rotating Protocol:

- Fenbendazole for 2-4 weeks
- Break for 1-2 weeks
- Mebendazole for 2-4 weeks
- Break for 1-2 weeks
- Repeat cycle

Lifestyle Factors

Don't forget non-pharmaceutical interventions:

Exercise:

- Improves outcomes in many cancers
- Reduces fatigue
- Enhances quality of life

- Supports immune function

Stress Management:

- Meditation or mindfulness
- Yoga or tai chi
- Counseling or support groups
- Adequate sleep

Social Support:

- Family and friends
- Support groups
- Online communities
- Spiritual practices

Sleep:

- 7-9 hours nightly
- Good sleep hygiene
- Address sleep disorders
- May use melatonin

Avoiding Harmful Exposures:

- No smoking
- Limit alcohol
- Avoid known carcinogens

- Reduce toxin exposure

Key Takeaways

- Many patients combine fenbendazole with supplements, repurposed drugs, dietary changes, and conventional treatments
- The Joe Tippens Protocol (fenbendazole + vitamin E + curcumin + CBD) is the most famous combination
- Rationale for combinations includes multiple mechanisms, potential synergy, and overcoming resistance
- Common additions include berberine, metformin, vitamin D, omega-3s, and various dietary approaches
- Integration with conventional treatment is most important but requires careful coordination with oncologists
- Timing strategies may reduce interactions and optimize effects
- Some combinations may be synergistic, while others could be antagonistic
- High-dose antioxidants during chemotherapy/radiation are controversial
- Safety considerations increase with each additional intervention—more monitoring needed
- Start simple, add gradually, document everything, and re-

assess regularly

- Work closely with your healthcare team when considering combinations
- Lifestyle factors (exercise, stress management, sleep) are important but often overlooked
- Complexity can reduce adherence—simpler may be better
- Most combinations lack scientific evidence—you're experimenting on yourself
- Quality of life and sustainability matter—don't make yourself miserable with too many interventions

PART FOUR: DECISION-MAKING FRAMEWORKS

Making decisions about unproven treatments like fenbendazole is challenging. You're facing uncertainty, conflicting information, emotional pressure, and potentially life-or-death stakes. This section provides frameworks to help you think through these difficult decisions systematically and thoughtfully.

CHAPTER TWELVE: MAKING YOUR OWN DECISION

Should you try fenbendazole? This is ultimately a personal decision that only you can make. This chapter provides a framework for thinking through this decision systematically, considering all relevant factors, and arriving at a choice you can feel confident about.

The Nature of the Decision

First, let's be clear about what kind of decision this is:

It's a Decision Under Uncertainty:

- We don't know if fenbendazole works for human cancer
- We don't know the optimal dose
- We don't know long-term effects

- We're making decisions with incomplete information

It's a Personal Decision:

- What's right for one person may not be right for another
- Your values, circumstances, and preferences matter
- There's no objectively "correct" answer
- You have to live with the consequences

It's a Medical Decision:

- It affects your health
- It interacts with other treatments
- It requires medical monitoring
- Healthcare professionals should be involved

It's a Reversible Decision:

- You can start and stop
- You can adjust your approach
- You can change your mind
- It's not all-or-nothing

It's Part of a Larger Strategy:

- Fenbendazole is one piece of your cancer treatment
- It should complement, not replace, proven treatments
- It fits into your overall approach to health

A Decision-Making Framework

Here's a systematic approach to making this decision:

Step 1: Clarify Your Situation

Your Cancer:

- Type and stage
- Prognosis with standard treatment
- Treatment options available
- Current treatment status

Your Health:

- Overall health status
- Other medical conditions
- Current medications
- Liver and kidney function

Your Circumstances:

- Financial resources
- Access to healthcare
- Support system
- Time and energy

Step 2: Define Your Goals

What are you hoping to achieve?

Possible Goals:

- Cure or remission
- Slow disease progression
- Extend survival
- Improve quality of life
- Reduce symptoms
- Enhance conventional treatment
- Feel like you're doing everything possible
- Maintain hope

Prioritize Your Goals:

- Which are most important?
- Which are realistic?
- Which are measurable?

Step 3: Gather Information

You've read this book, which is a good start. Also consider:

Scientific Evidence:

- Laboratory research
- Animal studies
- Lack of human trials
- Mechanisms of action

Patient Experiences:

- Anecdotal reports
- Online communities
- Limitations of anecdotes

Expert Opinions:

- Your oncologist's perspective
- Other doctors' views
- Scientific experts

Your Own Research:

- Scientific papers
- Reputable sources
- Critical evaluation

Step 4: Identify Your Options

What are your choices?

Option 1: Try Fenbendazole

- With conventional treatment
- Alone (if no other options)
- With other complementary approaches

Option 2: Don't Try Fenbendazole

- Focus on conventional treatment
- Try other complementary approaches
- Focus on quality of life

Option 3: Wait and See

- Monitor research developments
- Revisit decision later
- Try if conventional treatment fails

Option 4: Participate in Research

- Look for clinical trials
- Contribute to systematic data collection
- Help advance knowledge

Step 5: Evaluate Each Option

For each option, consider:

Potential Benefits:

- What's the best-case scenario?
- How likely is it?
- What evidence supports it?

Potential Risks:

- What's the worst-case scenario?
- How likely is it?
- What evidence suggests risks?

Costs:

- Financial costs
- Time and effort

- Emotional costs
- Opportunity costs

Alignment with Goals:

- Does this option serve your goals?
- How well does it fit your priorities?

Alignment with Values:

- Does this feel right to you?
- Is it consistent with your beliefs?
- Can you live with this choice?

Step 6: Consider Your Values

Your values should guide your decision:

Autonomy:

- How important is making your own choices?
- Do you want to take an active role?
- How do you feel about experimentation?

Evidence Standards:

- How much evidence do you need?
- Are you comfortable with uncertainty?
- Do you trust anecdotal reports?

Risk Tolerance:

- Are you risk-averse or risk-seeking?

- How do you weigh potential benefits vs. risks?
- What level of uncertainty can you tolerate?

Hope vs. Realism:

- How important is maintaining hope?
- How do you balance hope with realism?
- Can you accept uncertainty?

Quality vs. Quantity of Life:

- What matters more to you?
- How do you define quality of life?
- What trade-offs are acceptable?

Trust in Medicine:

- How much do you trust conventional medicine?
- How do you view alternative approaches?
- Where do you find credible information?

Step 7: Consult with Others

Don't make this decision in isolation:

Healthcare Team:

- Discuss with your oncologist
- Get input from other doctors
- Consider their expertise and concerns

Family and Friends:

- Discuss with loved ones
- Consider their perspectives
- They'll be affected by your decision

Other Patients:

- Learn from others' experiences
- Join support groups
- Get practical advice

Trusted Advisors:

- Spiritual counselors
- Therapists
- Others you trust

Step 8: Make a Provisional Decision

Based on all the above, make a tentative decision:

If Leaning Toward Trying Fenbendazole:

- What protocol will you use?
- How will you monitor?
- What's your plan for side effects?
- How long will you try it?
- What would make you stop?

If Leaning Against Trying Fenbendazole:

- What will you do instead?

- Are you comfortable with this choice?
- What would make you reconsider?

If Uncertain:

- What additional information do you need?
- What would help you decide?
- Is waiting an option?

Step 9: Test Your Decision

Before finalizing, test your decision:

The Regret Test:

- Imagine your cancer progresses. Would you regret not trying fenbendazole?
- Imagine fenbendazole causes problems. Would you regret trying it?
- Which regret would be harder to live with?

The Explanation Test:

- Can you explain your decision to others?
- Does your reasoning make sense?
- Are you comfortable defending your choice?

The Gut Check:

- How does this decision feel?
- Does it align with your intuition?
- Do you feel at peace with it?

The Reversibility Test:

- Can you change your mind later?
- What would trigger a change?
- Are you locked in or flexible?

Step 10: Implement and Reassess

Once you've decided:

If Trying Fenbendazole:

- Start with a clear protocol
- Establish monitoring plan
- Set decision points for reassessment
- Document everything

If Not Trying Fenbendazole:

- Focus on your chosen approach
- Don't second-guess constantly
- Revisit decision periodically
- Stay open to changing your mind

Regular Reassessment:

- Review your decision monthly
- Consider new information
- Evaluate whether it's working
- Adjust as needed

Common Decision-Making Pitfalls

Avoid these common mistakes:

Emotional Decision-Making:

- Deciding based on fear or desperation
- Not thinking clearly
- Ignoring rational considerations

Solution: Take time, calm down, use systematic framework

Analysis Paralysis:

- Overthinking to the point of inaction
- Waiting for perfect information
- Never feeling ready to decide

Solution: Set a decision deadline, accept uncertainty

Following the Crowd:

- Doing what others do without thinking
- Assuming others know better
- Not considering your unique situation

Solution: Make your own decision based on your circumstances

Ignoring Expert Advice:

- Dismissing doctors' concerns
- Thinking you know better
- Not seeking professional input

Solution: Listen to experts, even if you ultimately disagree

Confirmation Bias:

- Only seeking information that supports what you want to believe
- Ignoring contradictory evidence
- Rationalizing your preferred choice

Solution: Actively seek opposing viewpoints

Sunk Cost Fallacy:

- Continuing because you've already invested time/money
- Not wanting to admit it's not working
- Escalating commitment

Solution: Evaluate based on current situation, not past investment

Black-and-White Thinking:

- Seeing only two extreme options
- Missing middle ground
- All-or-nothing mentality

Solution: Consider nuanced approaches, partial measures

Special Considerations

Some situations require additional thought:

If You Have Limited Treatment Options:

- Fenbendazole may be more appealing
- Risk-benefit ratio shifts

- Less to lose by trying

If You Have Good Treatment Options:

- Focus on proven treatments first
- Fenbendazole as addition, not replacement
- Don't jeopardize effective treatment

If You're Doing Well:

- Consider whether to add fenbendazole
- "If it ain't broke, don't fix it" vs. "maximize every advantage"
- Maintenance approach

If You're Declining:

- May be willing to try anything
- Balance hope with quality of life
- Consider what matters most now

If You're Young:

- More years at stake
- May be more willing to experiment
- Long-term unknowns matter more

If You're Older:

- Different risk-benefit calculation
- Quality of life may be priority
- Shorter time horizon

If You Have Dependents:

- Consider impact on family
- Financial implications
- Time and energy for family

If You're Alone:

- Need for support system
- Who will help monitor?
- Who will advocate if problems arise?

Making Peace with Uncertainty

The hardest part of this decision is accepting uncertainty:

We Don't Know If It Works:

- No guarantees either way
- You're taking a chance
- Outcome is unpredictable

We Don't Know If It's Safe Long-Term:

- Unknown risks
- You're accepting this uncertainty
- Monitoring helps but doesn't eliminate risk

We Don't Know the Optimal Approach:

- Dose, schedule, duration all uncertain

- You're figuring it out as you go
- No roadmap to follow

Accepting Uncertainty:

- Acknowledge what we don't know
- Make the best decision you can with available information
- Be comfortable with "good enough" rather than perfect
- Trust your judgment
- Be willing to adjust

Finding Peace:

- Focus on your decision-making process, not the outcome
- You can only control your choices, not results
- Make a decision you can live with
- Let go of what you can't control

A Note on Hope

Hope is important, but it needs to be balanced:

Realistic Hope:

- Hope for the best
- Prepare for various outcomes
- Stay engaged with life

- Find meaning regardless of outcome

False Hope:

- Ignoring reality
- Magical thinking
- Refusing to consider alternatives
- Putting all eggs in one basket

Maintaining Hope While Being Realistic:

- Hope that fenbendazole might help
- Recognize it might not
- Have backup plans
- Find hope in multiple sources, not just one treatment

Your Decision Is Valid

Whatever you decide, your decision is valid if:

- You've thought it through carefully
- You've considered relevant information
- You've consulted with appropriate people
- It aligns with your values and goals
- You can live with the consequences
- You're willing to reassess

You don't need anyone's permission or approval. This is your life, your body, your decision.

Key Takeaways

- Deciding whether to try fenbendazole is a personal decision under uncertainty
- Use a systematic framework: clarify situation, define goals, gather information, identify options, evaluate each, consider values, consult others, make provisional decision, test it, implement and reassess
- Your values should guide your decision—there's no objectively "right" answer
- Avoid common pitfalls: emotional decision-making, analysis paralysis, following the crowd, ignoring experts, confirmation bias, sunk cost fallacy
- Special considerations apply based on your specific situation (treatment options, age, dependents, etc.)
- Accept uncertainty—we don't know if fenbendazole works, if it's safe long-term, or what the optimal approach is
- Balance hope with realism—hope for the best while preparing for various outcomes
- Your decision is valid if you've thought it through carefully and it aligns with your values
- This is a reversible decision—you can change your mind and

adjust your approach

- Regular reassessment is important—review your decision monthly and adjust as needed
- Make peace with uncertainty and focus on your decision-making process, not just the outcome
- Whatever you decide, you have the right to make your own informed choice

CHAPTER THIRTEEN: SPECIAL POPULATIONS

While most of this book addresses adult cancer patients generally, some populations have unique considerations. This chapter discusses fenbendazole use in children, elderly patients, pregnant or breastfeeding women, and other special situations.

Important Note: These populations are at higher risk and require even more caution. Everything in this chapter is informational, not medical advice. Specialized medical consultation is essential.

Pediatric Patients (Children and Adolescents)

Using fenbendazole in children with cancer raises unique concerns:

Why Pediatric Cancer Is Different:

Biological Differences:

- Children's bodies metabolize drugs differently
- Developing organs may be more vulnerable

- Growth and development considerations
- Different cancer types than adults

Treatment Differences:

- Pediatric cancers often more treatable than adult cancers
- Different chemotherapy protocols
- Higher cure rates for many pediatric cancers
- Long-term survivorship issues

Ethical Considerations:

- Children can't consent for themselves
- Parents make decisions
- Higher standard for safety
- Greater concern about long-term effects

Special Concerns for Fenbendazole in Children:

Lack of Data:

- No studies in children
- Unknown effects on development
- Unknown appropriate dosing
- Unknown long-term consequences

Dosing Challenges:

- Adult doses may not translate to children
- Weight-based dosing uncertain

- Age-related metabolism differences

Developmental Concerns:

- Effects on growing organs
- Impact on brain development
- Hormonal effects
- Long-term consequences

Higher Stakes:

- More years of life at stake
- Long-term effects matter more
- Cure rates often good with standard treatment
- Risk of jeopardizing proven treatments

When Might Fenbendazole Be Considered in Children:

Relapsed/Refractory Disease:

- When standard treatments have failed
- Limited other options
- Palliative situation
- After thorough discussion with pediatric oncologist

Rare Cancers:

- When no standard treatment exists
- Experimental situation anyway
- As part of compassionate use

Parental Decision:

- Parents have right to make informed decisions
- After full disclosure of unknowns
- With medical supervision
- Documenting decision-making process

Practical Considerations:

Dosing:

- Weight-based calculation from adult doses
- Start with lower end of range
- Increase gradually if tolerated
- Close monitoring

Formulation:

- Compounded capsules may be preferable
- Accurate dosing essential
- Taste considerations
- Ease of administration

Monitoring:

- More frequent than adults
- Growth and development tracking
- Careful attention to side effects
- Coordination with pediatric oncology team

Psychological Considerations:

- Age-appropriate explanation
- Child's assent (if old enough)
- Family support
- Coping with uncertainty

Recommendations for Parents:

1. **Prioritize Proven Treatments**: Don't let fenbendazole interfere with effective standard treatment
2. **Consult Pediatric Oncologist**: Essential for safety and coordination
3. **Consider Clinical Trials**: May offer better options than unproven treatments
4. **Document Everything**: Keep detailed records
5. **Support Your Child**: Emotional and psychological support crucial
6. **Connect with Other Families**: Pediatric cancer support groups
7. **Think Long-Term**: Consider effects on development and future health
8. **Be Prepared to Stop**: If any concerning effects

Elderly Patients (65+)

Older adults have different considerations:

Why Age Matters:

Physiological Changes:

- Decreased liver and kidney function
- Altered drug metabolism
- Multiple medical conditions
- Polypharmacy (many medications)

Different Goals:

- Quality of life may be priority
- Shorter life expectancy
- Different risk-benefit calculation
- Functional status important

Treatment Tolerance:

- May tolerate treatments less well
- Recovery slower
- Side effects more impactful
- Frailty considerations

Special Considerations for Elderly:

Reduced Drug Clearance:

- Liver and kidney function decline with age
- Drugs stay in system longer

- Lower doses may be appropriate
- More frequent monitoring needed

Drug Interactions:

- Elderly often take multiple medications
- Increased interaction risk
- Need comprehensive medication review
- Coordination with all doctors

Cognitive Considerations:

- Memory issues may affect adherence
- Understanding complex protocols
- Decision-making capacity
- Need for caregiver support

Functional Status:

- Ability to tolerate side effects
- Impact on daily activities
- Fall risk
- Independence considerations

When Fenbendazole Might Be Appropriate:

Good Functional Status:

- Active, independent elderly
- Good organ function

- Tolerating other treatments well
- Motivated to try

Limited Treatment Options:

- When standard treatments too toxic
- Palliative situation
- Quality of life focus

Informed Decision:

- Clear understanding of unknowns
- Realistic expectations
- Family support
- Medical supervision

Practical Considerations:

Dosing:

- Consider starting at lower dose
- Increase gradually
- Adjust based on kidney/liver function
- Monitor closely

Monitoring:

- More frequent blood tests
- Watch for drug interactions
- Assess functional status

- Cognitive monitoring

Simplification:

- Keep protocol simple
- Easy-to-follow schedule
- Pill organizers
- Caregiver assistance if needed

Coordination:

- Communicate with all doctors
- Comprehensive medication review
- Avoid duplicate testing
- Integrated care plan

Recommendations for Elderly Patients:

1. **Assess Functional Status**: Are you healthy enough to try this?
2. **Review All Medications**: Check for interactions
3. **Start Low, Go Slow**: Lower initial dose, gradual increases
4. **Simplify Protocol**: Don't overcomplicate
5. **Ensure Support**: Family or caregiver involvement
6. **Prioritize Quality of Life**: Don't sacrifice comfort for unproven treatment
7. **Regular Reassessment**: Is it worth continuing?

8. **Advance Planning**: Discuss goals of care

Pregnant or Breastfeeding Women

Pregnancy and breastfeeding create unique situations:

Pregnancy Considerations:

Fetal Risk:

- Benzimidazoles can cause birth defects in animals
- Fenbendazole crosses placenta
- Critical periods of development
- Unknown human effects

Recommendation:

- **Avoid fenbendazole during pregnancy unless absolutely necessary**
- Risk likely outweighs benefit in most cases
- Discuss with maternal-fetal medicine specialist
- Consider delaying treatment if possible

If Cancer Diagnosed During Pregnancy:

Timing Matters:

- First trimester most critical for development
- Some treatments safer in second/third trimester
- Delivery timing considerations

Difficult Decisions:

- Mother's life vs. fetal risk
- Termination considerations
- Delayed treatment risks
- Multidisciplinary consultation essential

If Fenbendazole Considered:

- Only in dire circumstances
- After thorough counseling
- Maternal-fetal medicine involvement
- Careful monitoring
- Informed consent

Breastfeeding Considerations:

Unknown Excretion:

- Don't know if fenbendazole enters breast milk
- Likely does to some degree
- Potential infant exposure

Recommendation:

- **Avoid fenbendazole while breastfeeding**
- Consider formula feeding if fenbendazole necessary
- Discuss with pediatrician
- Pump and dump if temporary

Fertility Considerations:

Unknown Effects:

- Impact on fertility unknown
- Effects on sperm or eggs unknown
- Pregnancy planning considerations

Recommendations:

- Use contraception while taking fenbendazole
- Discuss family planning with oncologist
- Consider fertility preservation before cancer treatment
- Wait period after stopping before attempting pregnancy

Patients with Liver Disease

Liver function is crucial for fenbendazole metabolism:

Why Liver Disease Matters:

Drug Metabolism:

- Liver metabolizes fenbendazole
- Impaired liver can't process drugs normally
- Drug accumulation risk
- Increased toxicity

Baseline Compromise:

- Liver already stressed

- Less reserve capacity
- Higher risk of liver damage

Considerations:

Mild Liver Disease:

- May be acceptable with close monitoring
- Reduced dose may be appropriate
- Frequent liver function tests
- Watch for worsening

Moderate to Severe Liver Disease:

- High risk
- Generally not recommended
- Only if benefits clearly outweigh risks
- Hepatologist consultation

Monitoring:

- Baseline liver function tests
- Frequent monitoring (weekly initially)
- Watch for signs of worsening
- Stop if liver enzymes rise significantly

Patients with Kidney Disease

Kidney function affects drug clearance:

Why Kidney Disease Matters:

Drug Clearance:

- Kidneys eliminate drugs and metabolites
- Impaired kidneys can't clear normally
- Drug accumulation possible

Considerations:

Mild Kidney Disease:

- Probably acceptable with monitoring
- May need dose adjustment
- Monitor kidney function

Moderate to Severe Kidney Disease:

- Increased caution
- Dose reduction likely needed
- Nephrologist consultation
- Close monitoring

Dialysis Patients:

- Unknown if dialysis removes fenbendazole
- Timing considerations
- Nephrologist must be involved

Patients with Compromised Immune Systems

Immune status affects cancer treatment:

Immunocompromised Patients:

Causes:

- HIV/AIDS
- Organ transplant (on immunosuppressants)
- Autoimmune disease treatments
- Chemotherapy effects

Concerns:

- Infection risk already elevated
- Unknown effects on immune function
- Drug interactions with immunosuppressants
- Complicated medical situation

Considerations:

- Infectious disease specialist consultation
- Close monitoring for infections
- Careful attention to drug interactions
- Risk-benefit assessment

Patients with Multiple Medical Conditions

Complex medical situations require extra caution:

Polypharmacy:

- Multiple medications increase interaction risk
- Comprehensive medication review essential
- Pharmacist consultation helpful

Multiple Organ Systems:

- Heart disease
- Lung disease
- Diabetes
- Others

Coordination:

- All specialists should be informed
- Integrated care plan
- Clear communication
- Avoid conflicting advice

Patients in Palliative or Hospice Care

End-of-life considerations are different:

Goals of Care:

- Comfort and quality of life priority
- Symptom management
- Time with loved ones

- Dignity and peace

Fenbendazole in Palliative Care:

Potential Role:

- If it provides hope without burden
- If side effects minimal
- If patient wants to try
- If it doesn't interfere with comfort

Potential Problems:

- May cause side effects that reduce comfort
- May give false hope
- May distract from important end-of-life issues
- May burden family

Considerations:

- What are patient's goals?
- Is this consistent with those goals?
- Does it enhance or detract from quality of life?
- What does patient truly want?

Honest Conversations:

- Realistic expectations
- Focus on what matters most
- Permission to stop trying

- Support for patient's choices

Cultural and Religious Considerations

Cultural and religious beliefs affect medical decisions:

Diverse Perspectives:

- Different cultures view illness differently
- Religious beliefs about treatment
- Traditional medicine practices
- Family decision-making structures

Respect and Sensitivity:

- Honor patient's beliefs
- Understand cultural context
- Involve appropriate family members
- Seek cultural competence

Integration:

- Fenbendazole may fit some belief systems
- May conflict with others
- Discuss openly
- Find common ground

Key Takeaways

- Special populations require extra caution and specialized medical consultation
- **Pediatric patients**: Higher risk, unknown developmental effects, only consider when standard treatments have failed, pediatric oncologist essential
- **Elderly patients**: Altered metabolism, multiple medications, start low and go slow, prioritize quality of life
- **Pregnant women**: Avoid fenbendazole—risk of birth defects, only in dire circumstances with specialist consultation
- **Breastfeeding women**: Avoid fenbendazole or stop breastfeeding, unknown excretion in milk
- **Liver disease**: Increased risk of toxicity, close monitoring essential, may need dose reduction or avoidance
- **Kidney disease**: May need dose adjustment, monitor kidney function, nephrologist consultation for severe disease
- **Immunocompromised**: Extra caution, specialist consultation, monitor for infections
- **Multiple medical conditions**: Comprehensive medication review, coordination among specialists, integrated care plan
- **Palliative/hospice care**: Focus on quality of life, realistic expectations, honest conversations about goals
- **Cultural/religious considerations**: Respect beliefs, cul-

tural sensitivity, involve appropriate family members

- All special populations need more frequent monitoring and closer medical supervision
- Risk-benefit calculations differ for special populations
- When in doubt, consult specialists familiar with the specific population

PART FIVE: LOOKING FORWARD

While this book has focused on what we know now about fenbendazole and cancer, it's important to look ahead. What research is needed? How can patients contribute? What does the future hold? This section explores these questions.

CHAPTER FOURTEEN: THE FUTURE OF FENBENDAZOLE RESEARCH

The fenbendazole story is far from over. While we lack clinical trial data now, that could change. This chapter explores what research is needed, barriers to conducting it, potential pathways forward, and how patients can contribute to advancing knowledge.

What Research Is Needed

To truly understand fenbendazole's potential in cancer treatment, we need:

Phase I Clinical Trials (Safety and Dosing):

Purpose:

- Establish safe dose range in humans
- Identify side effects
- Determine pharmacokinetics (how body processes drug)
- Find maximum tolerated dose

Design:

- Small number of patients (20-40)
- Dose escalation study
- Patients with advanced cancer
- Careful monitoring

What We'd Learn:

- What dose is safe?
- What side effects occur?
- How is it metabolized?
- What blood levels are achieved?

Phase II Clinical Trials (Preliminary Efficacy):

Purpose:

- Determine if fenbendazole shows anti-cancer activity
- Identify which cancer types respond
- Refine dosing
- Assess response rates

Design:

- 40-100 patients
- Specific cancer types
- Standardized dosing
- Objective response measurement

What We'd Learn:

- Does it show any activity?
- Which cancers respond?
- What's the response rate?
- What's the optimal dose?

Phase III Clinical Trials (Definitive Efficacy):

Purpose:

- Prove fenbendazole improves outcomes
- Compare to standard treatment
- Establish survival benefit
- Determine cost

Design:

- Hundreds to thousands of patients
- Randomized controlled trial
- Fenbendazole + standard care vs. standard care alone
- Multiple cancer centers

- Long-term follow-up (years)
- Objective endpoints (survival, progression-free survival, quality of life)

What We'd Learn:

- Does fenbendazole extend survival?
- By how much?
- Does it improve quality of life?
- What are long-term side effects?
- Is it cost-effective?
- Which patient populations benefit most?

Phase IV Trials (Post-Market Surveillance):

If fenbendazole were approved for cancer treatment, Phase IV studies would monitor:

- Long-term safety in large populations
- Rare side effects that didn't appear in smaller trials
- Real-world effectiveness outside controlled trial settings
- Optimal use in different patient populations
- Drug interactions in diverse patient groups

However, we're nowhere near Phase IV—we haven't even started Phase I.

Current Research Efforts

So what research is actually happening now?

Academic Interest:

Several research groups have published laboratory and animal studies on fenbendazole and cancer. These continue sporadically, driven by scientific curiosity rather than commercial interest. Recent publications include:

- Mechanistic studies exploring how fenbendazole affects cancer cells
- Combination studies with other drugs
- Studies in additional cancer types
- Investigation of optimal dosing and scheduling

Patient Registries:

Some researchers and patient advocates are attempting to create registries to systematically track patients using fenbendazole:

- Collecting baseline information
- Following outcomes over time
- Documenting side effects
- Analyzing patterns

These efforts face challenges including funding, patient recruitment, and data quality, but they represent important steps toward better evidence.

Crowdsourced Data:

Online patient communities are collecting informal data:

- Self-reported outcomes
- Dosing protocols
- Side effects
- Combination approaches

While not scientifically rigorous, this information provides insights into real-world use and could generate hypotheses for formal research.

International Efforts:

Some countries with different regulatory environments may be more open to fenbendazole research:

- Smaller pilot studies
- Compassionate use programs
- Integration with conventional treatment

However, no major clinical trials have been announced or initiated as of this writing.

Pharmaceutical Interest:

A few small companies have expressed interest in:

- Developing proprietary formulations of fenbendazole
- Conducting formal clinical trials
- Seeking regulatory approval

However, the economics remain challenging, and no trials have materialized.

Barriers to Research

Understanding why research hasn't progressed helps set realistic expectations:

Financial Barriers:

- Clinical trials cost $50-100 million
- No patent protection means no return on investment
- Pharmaceutical companies won't fund research on generic drugs
- Government funding agencies prioritize novel approaches
- Foundations focus on patentable innovations

Regulatory Barriers:

- FDA approval requires extensive data
- Fenbendazole is approved for veterinary use only
- Human use requires new approval process
- Liability concerns for researchers and institutions
- Complex regulatory pathway for repurposed drugs

Scientific Barriers:

- Limited preliminary human data
- Uncertainty about optimal dosing
- Unknown which cancer types might respond
- Difficulty designing trials without more information
- Academic researchers focus on novel mechanisms

Cultural Barriers:

- Skepticism about "alternative" approaches
- Resistance to patient-driven research
- Professional risk for researchers
- Concern about legitimizing unproven treatments
- Tension between patient advocacy and scientific rigor

Potential Pathways Forward

Despite these barriers, several models could enable fenbendazole research:

Philanthropic Funding:

Wealthy individuals or foundations could fund trials:

- Patient advocacy groups raising money
- Crowdfunding campaigns
- Donations from interested parties
- Non-profit research organizations

Government Funding:

Government agencies could prioritize repurposed drug research:

- NIH grants for drug repurposing
- National Cancer Institute initiatives
- International research collaborations

- Public health research programs

Academic-Industry Partnerships:

Collaborations between universities and companies:

- Shared costs and expertise
- Academic rigor with industry resources
- Creative funding models
- Intellectual property arrangements

Adaptive Trial Designs:

Innovative trial designs could reduce costs:

- Smaller, more efficient trials
- Adaptive designs that adjust based on results
- Platform trials testing multiple drugs
- Real-world evidence studies

International Collaboration:

Multi-country efforts could:

- Share costs across institutions
- Leverage different regulatory environments
- Pool patient populations
- Combine resources and expertise

Patient-Funded Research:

Patients themselves could fund research:

- Direct contributions to research funds

- Participation in data collection
- Advocacy for research funding
- Support for research infrastructure

How Patients Can Contribute to Research

Even without formal clinical trials, patients can contribute to advancing knowledge:

Participate in Registries:

If patient registries exist, consider enrolling:

- Provide baseline information
- Report outcomes honestly
- Document side effects
- Follow up consistently

Document Your Experience:

Keep detailed records:

- Treatment protocols
- Side effects
- Scan results
- Lab values
- Quality of life measures
- Concurrent treatments

This documentation could be valuable for future research.

Share Data Responsibly:

If you choose to share your experience:

- Be honest about outcomes (positive and negative)
- Provide complete information
- Avoid exaggeration or selective reporting
- Acknowledge uncertainties
- Respect others' privacy

Support Research Funding:

Consider supporting organizations working on:

- Repurposed drug research
- Patient-driven research initiatives
- Cancer research generally
- Open science efforts

Advocate for Research:

Use your voice to:

- Contact representatives about research funding
- Support policies enabling drug repurposing research
- Raise awareness about barriers to research
- Connect with patient advocacy organizations

Participate in Formal Studies:

If clinical trials eventually begin:

- Consider enrolling
- Spread the word to others
- Support trial recruitment
- Provide feedback to researchers

Maintain Scientific Rigor:

Help elevate the conversation:

- Distinguish evidence from anecdote
- Acknowledge uncertainties
- Avoid making unsupported claims
- Promote critical thinking
- Support evidence-based approaches

Timeline for Potential Clinical Trials

What's a realistic timeline for fenbendazole clinical trials?

Optimistic Scenario (5-7 years):

- Funding secured within 1-2 years
- Phase I trial designed and approved: 1 year
- Phase I conducted: 1-2 years
- Phase II designed and conducted: 2-3 years
- Results published and analyzed: 1 year

Realistic Scenario (10-15 years):

- Funding challenges delay start: 3-5 years
- Regulatory hurdles slow approval: 1-2 years
- Phase I: 2 years
- Phase II: 3-4 years
- Phase III (if warranted): 4-5 years
- Analysis and publication: 1-2 years

Pessimistic Scenario (Never):

- Funding never materializes
- No organization takes on the challenge
- Regulatory barriers prove insurmountable
- Scientific community remains uninterested
- Patient interest wanes

The honest answer is that we don't know. Clinical trials may never happen, or they could begin tomorrow if the right combination of funding, leadership, and circumstances aligns.

What This Means for Patients Now

The lack of clinical trials and uncertain research timeline has important implications:

You're Making Decisions Without Definitive Evidence:

If you choose to try fenbendazole, you're doing so based on:

- Laboratory research
- Animal studies
- Anecdotal reports
- Theoretical mechanisms
- Personal values and circumstances

This is not the same as making decisions based on clinical trial evidence.

The Evidence May Never Come:

It's possible that definitive evidence about fenbendazole and cancer will never be generated. You may need to make decisions in the face of permanent uncertainty.

You're Participating in an Uncontrolled Experiment:

By using fenbendazole, you're essentially conducting an experiment on yourself:

- No standardized protocol
- No systematic monitoring
- No control group
- No way to know if it's working
- No long-term safety data

Your Experience Matters:

Despite the limitations, your experience contributes to collective knowledge:

- It informs other patients' decisions

- It may generate hypotheses for research
- It demonstrates patient interest and need
- It could eventually lead to formal studies

Hope and Realism Must Coexist:

It's possible to:

- Hope that fenbendazole helps
- Acknowledge that we don't know if it does
- Make informed decisions despite uncertainty
- Contribute to knowledge while protecting yourself
- Maintain realistic expectations

Key Takeaways

- Proper clinical trials (Phase I-III) would take 5-15 years and cost $50-100 million
- No clinical trials of fenbendazole for cancer are currently underway or planned
- Barriers include lack of patent protection, regulatory hurdles, and limited funding
- Some academic research continues, and patient registries are being attempted
- Potential pathways forward include philanthropic funding,

government support, and innovative trial designs

- Patients can contribute by documenting experiences, participating in registries, and supporting research funding
- A realistic timeline for clinical trials is 10-15 years, if they happen at all
- Patients making decisions now must do so without clinical trial evidence and with the understanding that definitive evidence may never come
- The lack of trials doesn't mean fenbendazole doesn't work, but it means we can't know if it does
- Hope, realism, and informed decision-making must coexist in the face of uncertainty

CHAPTER FIFTEEN: THE BIGGER PICTURE

To understand the fenbendazole phenomenon, we need to step back and look at the broader landscape of cancer treatment, drug development, and the changing relationship between patients and medicine.

The Evolution of Cancer Treatment

Cancer treatment has evolved dramatically over the past century:

Surgery Era (early 1900s):

- Surgery was the only option
- Radical procedures were common
- Cure rates were low
- Quality of life often poor

Radiation Era (1920s-1950s):

- Radiation therapy emerged
- Combined with surgery
- Improved outcomes for some cancers
- Significant side effects

Chemotherapy Era (1950s-1990s):

- Systemic treatment became possible
- Combination chemotherapy improved cure rates
- Many cancers became treatable
- Toxicity remained a major challenge

Targeted Therapy Era (1990s-2010s):

- Drugs targeting specific molecular abnormalities
- Imatinib (Gleevec) revolutionized CML treatment
- HER2 inhibitors transformed breast cancer care
- More effective with fewer side effects than traditional chemotherapy

Immunotherapy Era (2010s-present):

- Checkpoint inhibitors unleash immune system
- CAR-T cell therapy for blood cancers
- Dramatic responses in some patients
- New paradigm for cancer treatment

Precision Medicine Era (emerging):

- Treatment based on tumor genetics
- Personalized therapy selection
- Liquid biopsies for monitoring
- AI-assisted treatment planning

Each era built on previous advances while introducing new possibilities and challenges.

Where Fenbendazole Fits

Fenbendazole represents something different from these established paradigms:

A Repurposed Drug:

Fenbendazole wasn't designed for cancer. It's a veterinary antiparasitic drug being explored for a completely different use. This is called "drug repurposing" or "drug repositioning."

Drug repurposing has precedents:

- Aspirin: Originally for pain, now used for heart disease prevention
- Thalidomide: Caused birth defects, now treats multiple myeloma
- Metformin: Diabetes drug, being studied for cancer prevention
- Viagra: Developed for heart disease, became erectile dysfunction treatment

Patient-Driven Discovery:

Unlike most cancer drugs, which are developed by pharmaceutical companies or academic researchers, fenbendazole's use in cancer emerged from:

- Accidental observation in a research lab
- One patient's dramatic response
- Viral spread through social media
- Patient experimentation and self-reporting

This bottom-up, patient-driven approach is relatively new in medicine.

Outside the System:

Fenbendazole exists outside the conventional drug development system:

- No pharmaceutical company backing
- No clinical trials
- No FDA approval for cancer
- No insurance coverage
- No standard protocols

This creates both opportunities (patient access, low cost) and challenges (no evidence, no guidance, no oversight).

The Repurposed Drug Challenge

Fenbendazole exemplifies a broader challenge in medicine: how do we study and integrate repurposed drugs?

The Economic Problem:

- Generic drugs can't be patented
- No patent means no exclusivity
- No exclusivity means no return on investment
- No return means no company will fund trials
- No trials means no evidence
- No evidence means no approval

This creates a "valley of death" where promising repurposed drugs languish despite potential benefits.

The Regulatory Problem:

- FDA approval requires extensive clinical trials
- Trials cost tens of millions of dollars
- Generic drugs don't generate revenue to justify costs
- Regulatory pathway for repurposed drugs is unclear
- Off-label use is legal but not officially supported

The Evidence Problem:

- Without trials, we can't know if repurposed drugs work
- Anecdotal reports are insufficient
- Patients use drugs without evidence

- Doctors can't recommend without evidence
- The cycle perpetuates

Potential Solutions:

Various stakeholders have proposed solutions:

- Government funding for repurposed drug trials
- Non-profit research organizations
- Adaptive trial designs to reduce costs
- Real-world evidence studies
- International collaboration
- Patient registries and observational studies

Some progress is being made, but the fundamental economic problem remains.

The Patient Empowerment Movement

Fenbendazole is part of a larger trend: patients taking more active roles in their healthcare.

Drivers of Patient Empowerment:

- Internet access to medical information
- Social media connecting patients
- Frustration with conventional medicine's limitations
- Desire for control in the face of serious illness

- Success stories inspiring others
- Distrust of pharmaceutical industry
- Rising healthcare costs

Benefits of Patient Empowerment:

- Patients become informed partners in care
- Patient experiences inform research
- Unmet needs become visible
- Innovation can come from unexpected sources
- Patients advocate for themselves and others

Risks of Patient Empowerment:

- Patients may make decisions based on poor information
- Anecdotes can be mistaken for evidence
- Desperation can lead to exploitation
- Unproven treatments may cause harm
- Patients may reject effective conventional treatments
- The burden of decision-making can be overwhelming

Finding Balance:

The goal is to empower patients while maintaining scientific rigor:

- Patients should have access to information
- But information should be accurate and contextualized

- Patients should have autonomy
- But with appropriate guidance and support
- Patient experiences matter
- But they must be distinguished from clinical evidence
- Innovation should be encouraged
- But safety and efficacy must be demonstrated

The Role of Uncertainty in Medicine

Fenbendazole highlights an uncomfortable truth: medicine involves more uncertainty than we often acknowledge.

Types of Uncertainty:

Scientific Uncertainty: We don't know if fenbendazole works for cancer

Personal Uncertainty: We don't know if it would work for you specifically

Practical Uncertainty: We don't know the optimal dose, schedule, or duration

Long-term Uncertainty: We don't know the long-term effects

Comparative Uncertainty: We don't know how it compares to other treatments

Living with Uncertainty:

Patients facing cancer must make decisions despite uncertainty:

- Which treatment to choose
- Whether to participate in clinical trials

- When to stop treatment
- How to balance quality and quantity of life
- Whether to try unproven approaches

Medicine's Response to Uncertainty:

The medical establishment typically responds to uncertainty with caution:

- Don't recommend treatments without evidence
- Emphasize proven approaches
- Warn against unproven treatments
- Wait for clinical trials

This is appropriate and protects patients from harm. But it can also feel dismissive to patients who are suffering now and can't wait for trials that may never come.

Patient Response to Uncertainty:

Patients often respond differently:

- Willing to try unproven treatments
- Accept risk in exchange for hope
- Value autonomy and choice
- Frustrated by "wait and see" approach
- Feel abandoned by conventional medicine

Neither response is wrong—they reflect different values, priorities, and positions.

Lessons from the Fenbendazole Story

What can we learn from the fenbendazole phenomenon?

For Patients:

- You have the right to make informed decisions about your care
- But "informed" means understanding both possibilities and limitations
- Anecdotes are not evidence, no matter how compelling
- Hope and realism can coexist
- Your healthcare team should be your partner, not your adversary
- Document your experiences—they may help others

For Healthcare Providers:

- Patients will explore options outside conventional medicine
- Dismissing their concerns damages trust
- Listening doesn't mean endorsing
- Harm reduction is better than prohibition
- Patients need guidance, not judgment
- Uncertainty is uncomfortable but honest

For Researchers:

- Patient interest signals unmet needs
- Repurposed drugs deserve more attention
- Creative funding models are needed
- Patient-reported data has value
- The perfect shouldn't be the enemy of the good
- Collaboration with patients can advance science

For the System:

- Current drug development models have gaps
- Repurposed drugs fall through the cracks
- Patient-driven research has a role
- Regulatory flexibility is needed
- Evidence standards must be maintained
- Innovation requires new approaches

The Future of Cancer Treatment

Where is cancer treatment heading, and where might fenbendazole fit?

Emerging Trends:

- Personalized medicine based on tumor genetics
- Immunotherapy combinations
- Metabolic approaches to cancer

- Repurposed drugs gaining attention
- Patient-generated data informing research
- AI and machine learning in treatment selection
- Liquid biopsies for early detection and monitoring

Potential Scenarios for Fenbendazole:

Scenario 1: Clinical Validation

- Trials are conducted and show benefit
- Fenbendazole becomes part of standard care
- Integrated with conventional treatments
- Protocols are established
- Patients have evidence-based option

Scenario 2: Niche Role

- Limited evidence emerges
- Some patients benefit, others don't
- Used in specific situations
- Remains somewhat controversial
- Accepted as one option among many

Scenario 3: Disproven

- Research shows no benefit
- Patient reports explained by other factors

- Interest wanes
- Remembered as a cautionary tale

Scenario 4: Perpetual Uncertainty

- No definitive research is conducted
- Anecdotal reports continue
- Patients keep using it
- Debate continues indefinitely
- We never know for sure

Currently, Scenario 4 seems most likely, though Scenarios 1-3 remain possible.

Hope, Hype, and Healing

The fenbendazole story involves all three:

Hope:

- Patients hoping for effective treatment
- Families hoping for more time with loved ones
- Researchers hoping to find new approaches
- Society hoping for cancer breakthroughs

Hope is essential. It motivates patients to keep fighting, researchers to keep searching, and families to keep supporting. Without hope, cancer would be unbearable.

Hype:

- Exaggerated claims about fenbendazole's effectiveness
- "Miracle cure" language
- Conspiracy theories about suppression
- Oversimplification of complex science
- Exploitation of desperate patients

Hype is dangerous. It creates false expectations, leads to poor decisions, and ultimately causes more suffering when reality doesn't match promises.

Healing:

- Physical healing from cancer
- Emotional healing from trauma
- Spiritual healing from suffering
- Relational healing with loved ones
- Existential healing through meaning-making

Healing is the goal, but it takes many forms. Sometimes healing means cure. Sometimes it means acceptance. Sometimes it means finding peace despite ongoing illness.

Distinguishing Among Them:

The challenge is maintaining hope without succumbing to hype, while remaining open to healing in all its forms:

- Hope grounded in reality
- Skepticism without cynicism

- Openness without gullibility
- Autonomy with guidance
- Action with acceptance

Key Takeaways

- Cancer treatment has evolved through multiple eras, each building on previous advances
- Fenbendazole represents a patient-driven, repurposed drug approach that exists outside conventional development systems
- The repurposed drug challenge involves economic, regulatory, and evidence problems with no easy solutions
- Patient empowerment has benefits and risks—the goal is informed autonomy with appropriate support
- Medicine involves more uncertainty than we often acknowledge, and different stakeholders respond to uncertainty differently
- The fenbendazole story offers lessons for patients, providers, researchers, and the healthcare system
- Future scenarios for fenbendazole range from clinical validation to perpetual uncertainty
- Hope, hype, and healing must be distinguished—hope is essential, hype is dangerous, healing takes many forms

- The fenbendazole phenomenon reflects broader tensions in medicine between innovation and evidence, autonomy and guidance, hope and realism

CHAPTER 16: FINAL THOUGHTS

As we near the end of this book, it's time to step back and reflect on what we've learned, what we haven't learned, and what it all means for you as you navigate your cancer journey.

What We Know

Let's summarize what we can say with confidence about fenbendazole and cancer:

Laboratory Evidence:

- Fenbendazole kills cancer cells in laboratory dishes
- It works through multiple mechanisms (microtubule disruption, metabolic interference, apoptosis)
- It shows activity against many cancer types in cell culture

- The concentrations that work in the lab are potentially achievable in humans

Animal Evidence:

- Fenbendazole slows tumor growth in mice
- It extends survival in some mouse cancer models
- It appears well-tolerated at doses that show anti-cancer effects
- It can be combined with conventional treatments in animals

Safety Profile:

- Fenbendazole has been used safely in animals for decades
- Veterinary use suggests a favorable safety profile
- Patient reports suggest it's generally well-tolerated
- Serious side effects appear rare but are not systematically documented

Mechanism:

- We understand how fenbendazole might work against cancer
- The mechanisms are biologically plausible
- They align with how other successful cancer drugs work

This is not nothing. This is a foundation that justifies interest and further investigation.

What We Don't Know

But the gaps in our knowledge are substantial:

Human Efficacy:

- We don't know if fenbendazole works in human cancer patients
- We don't know which cancer types might respond
- We don't know what percentage of patients might benefit
- We don't know how it compares to conventional treatments

Optimal Use:

- We don't know the best dose for humans
- We don't know the optimal schedule (daily, intermittent, pulsed)
- We don't know how long to use it
- We don't know the best formulation

Long-term Effects:

- We don't know the effects of years of use
- We don't know if resistance develops
- We don't know if there are cumulative toxicities
- We don't know long-term survival outcomes

Patient Selection:

- We don't know which patients are most likely to benefit
- We don't know if biomarkers could predict response

- We don't know if certain genetic profiles respond better

Combination Approaches:

- We don't know the best combinations with conventional treatment
- We don't know optimal timing and sequencing
- We don't know which combinations are synergistic vs. antagonistic

These unknowns are not trivial. They represent the difference between a proven treatment and an interesting possibility.

The Weight of Decision-Making

If you're considering fenbendazole, you're carrying a heavy burden: making a potentially life-or-death decision without adequate information.

This Isn't Fair:

You shouldn't have to make this decision. In an ideal world:

- Clinical trials would have been conducted
- Evidence would be available
- Doctors could provide clear guidance
- You could make informed decisions based on data

But we don't live in that world. The trials haven't been done, the evidence doesn't exist, and you must decide anyway.

You're Not Alone:

Thousands of cancer patients face similar decisions:

- Which treatment to choose among imperfect options
- Whether to participate in clinical trials
- When to stop treatment that isn't working
- Whether to try unproven approaches
- How to balance hope with realism

Cancer forces impossible decisions on people who are already suffering. This is one of the cruelties of the disease.

You're Doing Your Best:

Whatever you decide about fenbendazole:

- You're making the best decision you can with available information
- You're taking your health seriously
- You're advocating for yourself
- You're facing uncertainty with courage

Give yourself credit for that.

Permission to Choose

You need to hear this: you have permission to make your own decision about fenbendazole.

Permission to Try It:

If you decide to try fenbendazole:

- You're not being foolish
- You're not ignoring science

- You're not giving up on conventional medicine
- You're exercising informed autonomy

You have the right to try an unproven treatment if you understand the uncertainties and accept the risks.

Permission Not to Try It:

If you decide not to try fenbendazole:

- You're not giving up
- You're not being closed-minded
- You're not missing your only chance
- You're making a reasonable choice

You have the right to focus on proven treatments and not add unproven approaches to your regimen.

Permission to Change Your Mind:

If you try fenbendazole and later stop:

- You're not a quitter
- You're responding to new information
- You're adjusting your approach
- You're being flexible

If you initially decline but later decide to try it:

- You're not being inconsistent
- You're responding to changing circumstances
- You're remaining open

- You're adapting

Decisions about cancer treatment aren't permanent. You can adjust as you learn more about your disease, your response to treatment, and your priorities.

A Word About Hope

Hope is complicated in cancer care.

Hope Is Essential:

Without hope:

- Treatment becomes unbearable
- Life loses meaning
- Relationships suffer
- Quality of life plummets

Hope motivates patients to keep fighting, families to keep supporting, and researchers to keep searching for better treatments.

But Hope Can Be Dangerous:

When hope becomes:

- Denial of reality
- Rejection of proven treatments
- Vulnerability to exploitation
- Inability to prepare for difficult outcomes
- Source of crushing disappointment

Realistic Hope:

The goal is hope that's grounded in reality:

- Hope that fenbendazole might help, while acknowledging it might not
- Hope for more time, while accepting mortality
- Hope for quality of life, not just quantity
- Hope for meaning and connection, regardless of outcome
- Hope that coexists with preparation for various possibilities

Hope Is Not the Same as Expectation:

You can hope fenbendazole will help without expecting it to cure your cancer. You can hope for the best while preparing for various outcomes. You can maintain hope while also being realistic about probabilities.

This distinction is crucial. Expectation leads to devastation when things don't work out. Hope, properly calibrated, can sustain you through uncertainty without setting you up for crushing disappointment.

Living Fully in the Face of Uncertainty

Cancer forces you to live with uncertainty. Adding fenbendazole to your treatment adds another layer of uncertainty. How do you live fully when so much is unknown?

Focus on What You Can Control:

You cannot control:

- Whether fenbendazole will work
- How your cancer will progress

- How long you'll live
- Whether research will eventually prove fenbendazole effective

You can control:

- Your decision-making process
- How you treat yourself and others
- What you do with your time
- Your relationships and connections
- Your attitude toward uncertainty
- How you define quality of life

Find Meaning Beyond Outcomes:

Your life's meaning doesn't depend on whether fenbendazole works. Meaning comes from:

- Relationships and love
- How you face challenges
- What you learn and share
- How you treat others
- The legacy you create
- Living according to your values

Practice Acceptance:

Acceptance doesn't mean giving up. It means:

- Acknowledging reality as it is
- Letting go of what you cannot control
- Making peace with uncertainty
- Finding contentment despite circumstances
- Reducing suffering caused by resistance

Stay Present:

Uncertainty pulls you into the future—worrying about what might happen. But life happens now:

- This moment is all you truly have
- Quality of life is experienced in the present
- Relationships happen now
- Joy and meaning are found in the present

Build Resilience:

Resilience helps you navigate uncertainty:

- Develop coping strategies
- Build support networks
- Practice self-compassion
- Maintain flexibility
- Learn from challenges
- Find strength you didn't know you had

The Courage to Choose

Making decisions about unproven treatments requires courage. You're choosing despite uncertainty, despite conflicting advice, despite not knowing how things will turn out.

This courage deserves recognition. Whether you decide to try fenbendazole or not, whether it works or doesn't, you're facing one of life's most difficult challenges with bravery.

The Courage to Try:

If you decide to use fenbendazole, you're showing courage by:

- Taking responsibility for your health
- Accepting uncertainty
- Risking disappointment
- Going against conventional wisdom
- Advocating for yourself

The Courage Not to Try:

If you decide against fenbendazole, you're showing courage by:

- Accepting limitations
- Trusting proven approaches
- Resisting pressure from others
- Making peace with your choice
- Living with "what ifs"

Both choices require courage. Neither is the "right" choice for everyone.

A Message to Families and Caregivers

If you're reading this book to support someone considering fenbendazole, you face your own challenges:

Your Role:

- Support their decision-making process
- Provide information without pressure
- Respect their autonomy
- Help them think clearly
- Be present with their uncertainty

Your Challenges:

- You may disagree with their choice
- You may feel helpless
- You may struggle with your own hope and fear
- You may face criticism from others
- You may need to advocate for them

Your Needs Matter Too:

- Seek your own support
- Process your own emotions

- Set boundaries when needed
- Take care of yourself
- Find your own meaning in this experience

Remember:

- This is their journey, not yours
- Your job is to support, not control
- Love doesn't mean agreement
- You can disagree and still support
- Your presence matters more than your opinions

Moving Forward

As you close this book and move forward with your decision, remember:

You Are Not Alone:

Thousands of patients face similar decisions. Communities exist to support you. Healthcare providers, despite disagreements, want to help. You're part of a larger story of patients navigating uncertainty.

You Are Doing Your Best:

With the information available, the time you have, the resources you can access, and the support you can find—you're doing your best. That's all anyone can do.

Your Decision Is Valid:

Whatever you decide, if you've thought it through carefully, considered the evidence, consulted with others, and aligned your choice with your values—your decision is valid. You don't need anyone's permission or approval.

The Story Isn't Over:

Whether you try fenbendazole or not, your story continues. New information will emerge. Circumstances will change. You'll learn and adapt. The decision you make today isn't the end—it's part of an ongoing journey.

You Have Agency:

In a situation where so much is beyond your control, you have agency in how you respond. You can make informed choices. You can advocate for yourself. You can live according to your values. This agency is powerful and meaningful.

Final Reflections

The fenbendazole story is remarkable not because we know it works, but because it reveals something important about cancer care, medical research, and patient empowerment.

It shows us:

- The gap between laboratory promise and clinical proof
- The limitations of our current research funding models
- The power and limitations of patient-driven research
- The tension between evidence standards and patient needs
- The complexity of hope, autonomy, and uncertainty

Whether fenbendazole ultimately proves effective or not, this phenomenon has already contributed something valuable: it's sparked conversations about how we research treatments, how we support patient autonomy, and how we navigate uncertainty in medicine.

Your engagement with this question—reading this book, thinking critically, making informed decisions—is part of that contribution. You're not just a passive recipient of medical care. You're an active participant in your health, in medical knowledge, and in the ongoing evolution of how we approach cancer treatment.

A Closing Thought

Cancer is one of life's greatest challenges. It tests everything—your body, your mind, your relationships, your beliefs, your courage. There are no easy answers, no guaranteed solutions, no paths without risk.

But you don't have to have all the answers. You don't have to make perfect decisions. You don't have to face this alone.

What you need is:

- Good information (which you now have)
- Critical thinking (which you've practiced)
- Support from others (which you can seek)
- Compassion for yourself (which you deserve)
- Courage to choose (which you possess)

Whether fenbendazole becomes part of your cancer journey or not, whether it helps or doesn't, whether research eventually validates it or not—you are more than this decision. You are more than your cancer. You are a whole person navigating an impossibly difficult situation with courage, intelligence, and humanity.

That's what matters most.

Key Takeaways

- Living with uncertainty is inherent to cancer care, and adding fenbendazole increases that uncertainty
- You can make good decisions despite incomplete information by focusing on your process, not just outcomes
- Hope is essential but must be balanced with realism—hope for possibilities while preparing for various outcomes
- Focus on what you can control: your decision-making, relationships, values, and how you spend your time
- Meaning comes from how you live, not just from treatment outcomes
- Both choosing to try fenbendazole and choosing not to try require courage
- Your decision is valid if it's informed, thoughtful, and aligned with your values
- Families and caregivers have their own challenges and need support too
- You have agency in how you respond to cancer, even when much is beyond your control
- The fenbendazole phenomenon reveals important truths about medical research, patient empowerment, and navigating uncertainty

- You are more than this decision, more than your cancer—you are a whole person with inherent worth
- Whatever you decide, approach yourself with compassion and recognize the courage it takes to face cancer

CONCLUSION

This book began with Joe Tippens' remarkable story and a simple question: Could a veterinary deworming drug help treat human cancer?

After exploring the laboratory research, animal studies, patient reports, practical considerations, and ethical dimensions, we arrive not at a simple answer, but at a more nuanced understanding.

What We Know:

- Fenbendazole has demonstrated anti-cancer activity in laboratory cell cultures across multiple cancer types
- Animal studies show it can slow tumor growth and extend survival in mice
- The mechanisms by which it might work are scientifically plausible
- It appears relatively safe based on decades of veterinary use
- Thousands of cancer patients have used it, with many reporting positive experiences
- It's accessible and affordable compared to conventional cancer drugs

What We Don't Know:

- Whether it actually works in human cancer patients
- What dose is optimal for humans
- Which cancer types might respond
- How it compares to or interacts with standard treatments
- What the long-term effects are
- Who might benefit most
- Whether the anecdotal reports reflect real efficacy or other factors

The Gap Between:

The gap between what we know and what we need to know is substantial. This gap creates the central challenge: patients need answers now, but science moves slowly. The evidence is intriguing but incomplete. The need is urgent but the research is absent.

Your Path Forward:

If you're considering fenbendazole, you now have:

- A thorough understanding of the scientific rationale
- A realistic assessment of the evidence
- Practical guidance on sourcing, dosing, and monitoring
- Frameworks for making informed decisions
- Awareness of risks, uncertainties, and limitations
- Tools for working with your healthcare team

What you do with this information is up to you. This book cannot make your decision for you—nor should it. Your decision must be yours, informed by your values, circumstances, and priorities.

A Balanced Perspective:

Fenbendazole is neither a miracle cure nor a dangerous fraud. It's an intriguing possibility that deserves serious research but lacks the clinical evidence needed to prove it works. It represents both the promise of repurposed drugs and the challenges of studying them.

Patients who choose to try it are not foolish or desperate—they're making informed decisions in the face of uncertainty. Patients who choose not to try it are not closed-minded or passive—they're also making informed decisions based on their assessment of evidence and risk.

Doctors who are skeptical are not dismissive or paternalistic—they're upholding evidence standards that protect patients. Doctors who are open to it are not reckless or unprofessional—they're respecting patient autonomy while providing guidance.

The truth is complex, and reasonable people can reach different conclusions.

The Bigger Picture:

The fenbendazole story is about more than one drug. It's about:

- How we fund and conduct medical research
- How we balance evidence standards with patient needs
- How we respect patient autonomy while providing expert guidance
- How we navigate uncertainty in medicine
- How we support people facing life-threatening illness

These questions matter beyond fenbendazole. They affect how we approach all of cancer care, all of medicine, and all of healthcare decision-making.

Looking Ahead:

The fenbendazole story is still being written. Perhaps clinical trials will eventually be conducted. Perhaps they'll show it works, or perhaps they'll show it doesn't. Perhaps the answer will be more nuanced—it works for some cancers but not others, or it helps some patients but not all.

Or perhaps trials will never happen, and fenbendazole will remain in this liminal space between laboratory promise and clinical proof, used by some patients, dismissed by some doctors, and debated by all.

Whatever happens, the conversations this phenomenon has sparked—about research, evidence, autonomy, and hope—are valuable in themselves.

A Final Word:

If you're reading this because you or someone you love has cancer, you're facing one of life's greatest challenges. You're navigating impossible decisions with incomplete information. You're balancing hope and realism, autonomy and guidance, action and acceptance.

This is hard. It's supposed to be hard. There are no easy answers.

But you're not powerless. You can educate yourself. You can think critically. You can make informed decisions. You can advocate for yourself. You can live according to your values. You can find meaning and connection even in the midst of uncertainty.

Whether fenbendazole becomes part of your journey or not, you have the capacity to face this challenge with courage, wisdom, and humanity.

That's what this book has tried to support—not to tell you what to do, but to help you think clearly, decide wisely, and move forward with confidence in your ability to navigate this difficult terrain.

You've got this. Not because the path is easy or the outcome is certain, but because you have what it takes to face uncertainty with courage and make the best decisions you can with the information available.

And that, ultimately, is all any of us can do.

RESOURCES AND FURTHER READING

Scientific Databases and Research

PubMed (pubmed.ncbi.nlm.nih.gov)

- Free database of biomedical literature
- Search "fenbendazole cancer" for research papers
- Includes abstracts and some full-text articles

Google Scholar (scholar.google.com)

- Broader academic search engine
- Often finds free versions of papers
- Good for finding related research

ClinicalTrials.gov

- Database of clinical trials worldwide
- Check for any fenbendazole trials

- Find other trials you might be eligible for

Patient Communities and Information

Telegram Groups

- Various fenbendazole-focused groups exist
- Share experiences and practical information
- Exercise critical thinking with all information

Facebook Groups

- Multiple groups dedicated to fenbendazole and cancer
- Search "fenbendazole cancer" to find active communities
- Remember that anecdotes are not data

Cancer Support Organizations

- American Cancer Society (cancer.org)
- Cancer Support Community (cancersupportcommunity.org)
- National Cancer Institute (cancer.gov)

Books on Cancer and Treatment Decision-Making

- "The Emperor of All Maladies" by Siddhartha Mukherjee (cancer history and biology)
- "Being Mortal" by Atul Gawande (end-of-life care and deci-

sion-making)

- "The Death of Cancer" by Vincent DeVita (cancer treatment evolution)
- "Anticancer: A New Way of Life" by David Servan-Schreiber (lifestyle and cancer)

Understanding Medical Research

- "Bad Science" by Ben Goldacre (critical evaluation of medical claims)
- "The Truth About Drug Companies" by Marcia Angell (pharmaceutical industry)
- "Doctoring Data" by Malcolm Kendrick (understanding medical statistics)

Complementary and Integrative Oncology

Society for Integrative Oncology (integrativeonc.org)

- Evidence-based information on complementary approaches
- Find integrative oncology practitioners

Memorial Sloan Kettering Cancer Center (mskcc.org/cancer-care/diagnosis-treatment/symptom-management/integrative-medicine)

- About Herbs database

- Evidence-based information on supplements and herbs

Repurposed Drugs and Cancer

ReDO Project (redo-project.org)

- Repurposing Drugs in Oncology
- Scientific information on repurposed drugs
- Evidence summaries

Care Oncology Clinic (careoncologyclinic.com)

- Clinic using repurposed drugs
- Information on metformin, atorvastatin, mebendazole, doxycycline

Finding Clinical Trials

- ClinicalTrials.gov (primary U.S. database)
- Cancer.gov/about-cancer/treatment/clinical-trials (NCI trial information)
- EmergingMed.com (trial matching service)
- Your cancer center's clinical trials office

Second Opinion Resources

- National Cancer Institute Cancer Information Service:

1-800-4-CANCER

- Major cancer centers offer second opinion programs
- Many offer virtual second opinions

Financial Assistance

- Patient Advocate Foundation (patientadvocate.org)
- CancerCare (cancercare.org) - financial assistance and counseling
- Pharmaceutical company patient assistance programs
- Hospital financial counselors

Legal and Ethical Resources

Right to Try

- FDA information: fda.gov/patients/learn-about-expanded-access-and-other-treatment-options
- State-specific right to try laws

Patient Rights

- Patient Advocate Foundation
- Center for Patient Partnerships (law.wisc.edu/gls/cpp)

Caregiver Support

- Family Caregiver Alliance (caregiver.org)
- Cancer Support Community (for patients and caregivers)
- Local hospice organizations (provide support even before end-of-life)

Important Disclaimer

This resource list is provided for informational purposes only. Inclusion does not constitute endorsement. Always verify information from multiple sources and consult with qualified healthcare professionals.

GLOSSARY OF KEY TERMS

Anecdotal Evidence: Information based on personal accounts or observations rather than systematic research. While valuable for generating hypotheses, anecdotal evidence cannot prove causation or establish treatment efficacy.

Apoptosis: Programmed cell death. A normal process by which cells die in a controlled manner. Cancer treatments often work by triggering apoptosis in cancer cells.

Benzimidazole: A class of chemical compounds that includes fenbendazole and related drugs like mebendazole and albendazole. These compounds share a similar chemical structure.

Bioavailability: The proportion of a drug that enters circulation and can have an active effect. Fenbendazole has relatively low bioavailability, meaning only a portion of an oral dose reaches the bloodstream.

Case Report: A detailed report of a single patient's diagnosis, treatment, and outcome. Case reports can be interesting but cannot prove that a treatment works.

Case Series: A collection of case reports involving multiple patients. More informative than single cases but still cannot establish causation without controls.

Cell Culture: Growing cells in a laboratory dish. Cell culture studies are the first step in testing whether a drug has anti-cancer effects, but results don't always translate to living organisms.

Clinical Trial: A research study involving human participants designed to evaluate medical interventions. Clinical trials are the gold standard for proving whether treatments work.

Compounding Pharmacy: A pharmacy that creates customized medications, including making fenbendazole capsules for human use (requires prescription).

Confirmation Bias: The tendency to search for, interpret, and remember information that confirms pre-existing beliefs while discounting contradictory evidence.

Cytotoxic: Toxic to cells. Chemotherapy drugs are cytotoxic, killing both cancer cells and some normal cells.

Dose-Response Relationship: The relationship between the amount of a drug given and the magnitude of its effect. A clear dose-response relationship strengthens evidence that a drug is causing an observed effect.

Efficacy: The ability of a treatment to produce the desired effect under ideal conditions (as in a clinical trial). Different from effectiveness (real-world performance).

Fenbendazole: A benzimidazole anthelmintic drug used in veterinary medicine to treat parasitic worm infections. Chemical formula: C15H13N3O2S.

Glucose Transporter (GLUT): Proteins that transport glucose across cell membranes. Cancer cells often have elevated GLUT expression. Fenbendazole may interfere with glucose uptake.

Half-Life: The time it takes for half of a drug to be eliminated from the body. Fenbendazole's half-life in mice is approximately 10-15 hours.

In Vitro: Literally "in glass"—refers to studies conducted in laboratory dishes or test tubes (cell culture studies).

In Vivo: Literally "in life"—refers to studies conducted in living organisms (animal studies or human trials).

Informed Consent: The process by which patients receive information about risks and benefits of a treatment and voluntarily agree to proceed. Essential for ethical medical care.

Mechanism of Action: How a drug produces its effects at the molecular and cellular level. Fenbendazole's primary mechanism involves microtubule disruption.

Metabolite: A substance produced when the body breaks down (metabolizes) a drug. Some of fenbendazole's metabolites also have anti-cancer activity.

Metastasis: The spread of cancer from its original site to other parts of the body. Metastatic cancer is generally more difficult to treat than localized cancer.

Microtubules: Hollow tubes made of protein that form part of the cell's structural framework. They're essential for cell division. Fenbendazole disrupts microtubules, preventing cancer cells from dividing.

Mitosis: The process of cell division. Cancer cells divide uncontrollably. Drugs that disrupt mitosis can stop cancer growth.

Off-Label Use: Using an approved drug for a purpose not specified in its official approval. Common in medicine but means the use hasn't been specifically studied or approved.

Oncologist: A doctor who specializes in treating cancer. Medical oncologists manage chemotherapy and systemic treatments.

p53: A tumor suppressor protein often called the "guardian of the genome." It triggers cell death when DNA is damaged. Many cancers have mutated p53. Fenbendazole may work through p53-related pathways.

Palliative Care: Medical care focused on providing relief from symptoms and improving quality of life, regardless of whether curative treatment is being pursued.

Peer Review: The process by which scientific research is evaluated by other experts before publication. Helps ensure quality but doesn't guarantee correctness.

Pharmacokinetics: The study of how the body absorbs, distributes, metabolizes, and excretes drugs. Understanding pharmacokinetics helps determine appropriate dosing.

Phase I Trial: The first stage of testing a drug in humans, focused on safety and dosing rather than efficacy.

Phase II Trial: The second stage, testing whether a drug shows preliminary evidence of efficacy in a specific condition.

Phase III Trial: The definitive stage, comparing the new treatment to standard treatment in a large, randomized trial.

Placebo Effect: Improvement in symptoms or condition due to belief in a treatment rather than the treatment's specific effects. Real and measurable, but doesn't affect objective outcomes like tumor size.

Prognosis: The likely course and outcome of a disease. Prognosis helps patients and doctors make treatment decisions.

Randomized Controlled Trial (RCT): A study in which participants are randomly assigned to receive either the treatment being tested or a control (placebo or standard treatment). The gold standard for proving causation.

Repurposed Drug: A medication approved for one use that's being investigated or used for a different condition. Fenbendazole is being repurposed from veterinary antiparasitic to potential cancer treatment.

Selection Bias: A distortion in results that occurs when the sample studied is not representative of the population. In patient reports, selection bias occurs because people with positive outcomes are more likely to share their experiences.

Synergy: When two treatments work together to produce an effect greater than the sum of their individual effects. Some combinations may be synergistic.

Therapeutic Window: The range between the dose that produces therapeutic effects and the dose that produces toxic effects. A wide therapeutic window is desirable.

Tumor Microenvironment: The cellular environment in which a tumor exists, including blood vessels, immune cells, and other cells. The microenvironment affects how tumors grow and respond to treatment.

Warburg Effect: The observation that cancer cells preferentially use glycolysis (sugar metabolism) even when oxygen is available. Named after Otto Warburg. Fenbendazole may interfere with this metabolic preference.

Xenograft: A tumor from one species transplanted into another species, typically human cancer cells transplanted into mice. Used in cancer research to test treatments.

ACKNOWLEDGMENTS

This book would not have been possible without the contributions of many people, though any errors or shortcomings are entirely my own.

First and foremost, I am grateful to the cancer patients and families who have shared their experiences with fenbendazole. Your willingness to document your journeys, share your data, and support others facing similar decisions has created a valuable resource for the entire community. Whether your experiences were positive, negative, or uncertain, your honesty has helped others make more informed decisions.

Special acknowledgment goes to Joe Tippens, whose willingness to share his story publicly sparked the conversation that may have led to this book. Regardless of what future research reveals about fenbendazole's efficacy, your openness about your experience has empowered countless patients to take a more active role in their healthcare decisions.

I am indebted to the researchers whose laboratory and animal studies form the scientific foundation of this book. Your work—often conducted without fanfare or significant funding—has revealed intriguing possibilities that deserve further investigation. Special thanks to those scientists who have taken the time to explain their research to non-specialists and who have engaged thoughtfully with patient questions.

Thank you to the oncologists, nurses, and other healthcare professionals who have approached the fenbendazole question with open minds and compassionate hearts. Those of you who have supported patients' informed decisions, even when you couldn't recommend fenbendazole yourselves, exemplify the best of patient-centered care. Your willingness to monitor patients, order appropriate tests, and maintain therapeutic relationships despite disagreements about unproven treatments demonstrates true professionalism.

I am grateful to the online communities—on Facebook, Telegram, Reddit, and other platforms—where patients share information, support each other, and collectively navigate uncertainty. While these communities sometimes spread misinformation, they more often provide invaluable practical guidance, emotional support, and a sense of solidarity that the formal healthcare system cannot always offer.

Thank you to the advocates working to reform how we research and fund repurposed drugs. Your efforts to create new models for studying off-patent medications address a critical gap in our medical research system. The fenbendazole phenomenon highlights why this work matters.

I am grateful to the critical thinkers and skeptics who have questioned claims about fenbendazole and demanded higher standards of evidence. Your skepticism, when expressed constructively, helps protect patients from false hope and exploitation. The tension between hope and skepticism, properly balanced, leads to better decision-making.

Thank you to the family members and caregivers who support loved ones through cancer treatment, including those who support decisions they may not fully agree with. Your love, patience, and presence matter more than you know.

I am indebted to the writers, researchers, and thinkers whose work on medical decision-making, evidence evaluation, and patient autonomy informed this book. Your insights about navigating uncertainty in medicine provided the intellectual framework for approaching this complex topic.

Thank you to those who reviewed drafts of this manuscript and provided feedback—both those who thought I was too credulous about fenbendazole's potential and those who thought I was too skeptical. Your competing perspectives helped me find a more balanced approach.

I am grateful to the librarians and information specialists who maintain the databases and resources that made this research possible.

PubMed, Google Scholar, and other open-access resources democratize medical knowledge in ways that empower patients.

Finally, I acknowledge the fundamental uncertainty that permeates this topic. We don't know if fenbendazole works for human cancer. We don't know if it will ever be properly studied. We don't, yet we push ahead.

www.ingramcontent.com/pod-product-compliance
Lightning Source LLC
LaVergne TN
LVHW010601100826
845148LV00014B/2795